Ethics and Values for Care Workers

Ethics and Values for Care Workers

G.V. Tadd

b

Blackwell
Science

© 1998 by Blackwell Science Ltd
Editorial Offices:
Osney Mead, Oxford OX2 0EL
25 John Street, London WC1N 2BL
23 Ainslie Place, Edinburgh EH3 6AJ
350 Main Street, Malden
  MA 02148 5018, USA
54 University Street, Carlton
  Victoria 3053, Australia

Other Editorial Offices:

Blackwell Wissenschafts-Verlag GmbH
Kurfürstendamm 57
10707 Berlin, Germany

Blackwell Science KK
MG Kodenmacho Building
7-10 Kodenmacho Nihombashi
Chuo-ku, Tokyo 104, Japan

First published 1998

Set in 10.5/13.5 pt Sabon
by DP Photosetting, Aylesbury, Bucks
Printed and bound in Great Britain by
MPG Books Ltd, Bodmin, Cornwall

The Blackwell Science logo is a trade mark of
Blackwell Science Ltd, registered at the United
Kingdom Trade Marks Registry

DISTRIBUTORS

Marston Book Services Ltd
PO Box 269
Abingdon
Oxon OX14 4YN
(*Orders:* Tel: 01235 465500
            Fax: 01235 465555)

USA
Blackwell Science, Inc.
Commerce Place
350 Main Street
Malden, MA 02148 5018
(*Orders:* Tel: 800 759 6102
                  617 388 8250
            Fax: 617 388 8255)

Canada
Copp Clark Professional
200 Adelaide Street West, 3rd Floor
Toronto, Ontario M5H 1W7
(*Orders:* Tel: 416 597 1616
                 800 815 9417
            Fax: 416 597 1617)

Australia
Blackwell Science Pty Ltd
54 University Street
Carlton, Victoria 3053
(*Orders:* Tel: 03 9347 0300
            Fax: 03 9347 5001)

A catalogue record for this title is available
from the British Library

ISBN 0-632-04814-X

Library of Congress
Cataloging-in-Publication Data
Tadd, G. V.
    Ethics and values for care workers/by G.V.
    Tadd.
        p.   cm.
    Includes bibliographical references and
    index.
    ISBN 0-632-04814-X (pbk.)
    1. Long-term care of the sick – Moral and
ethical aspects.   2. Handicapped – Long-
term care – Moral and ethical aspects.
I. Title.
RT120.L64T33   1998
174′.2 – dc21   97-41491
                                         CIP

Contents

Introduction

The care sector is a major employer of staff in this country. This is a trend that is likely to continue as the life span of the population goes on increasing. In the future more people will need some form of social or health care at least some time in their lives. Consequently, opportunities for a career in the care sector are bright for people who are interested in this type of work.

It is important that people who work in the caring professions have a genuine concern for the welfare of their clients, and that they are committed to maintaining high standards of care. An understanding of ethics can help them in this endeavour, providing that it is seen, not as an obscure academic exercise, but as an integral part of daily practice.

The last decade has seen a large number of books written on the subject of health care ethics. Many of these have been targeted specifically at professionally qualified staff, such as doctors and nurses, despite the fact that the majority of health and social care in this country is provided by non-professional staff. By comparison, relatively little on this topic has been written for the needs of unqualified staff working in social services or the health sector.

This book seeks to address this oversight. It is written specifically for those employed, or wishing to work, in residential and nursing homes in the private, public or voluntary sector. The text focuses particularly upon the needs of vulnerable client groups, such as older people, people with learning disabilities or those with an associated mental illness.

The ethical incidents discussed are not those which are the normal stuff of media headlines. Nor are they usually subjects of grand philosophical debate. In the main, they are representative of the sort of everyday situations which care staff are likely to meet in their daily practice.

The book explains the meaning of ethics and why they are important. The meaning of ethical principles, such as autonomy, paternalism and justice, is also discussed, but the emphasis is on the practical application of ethics and theory is kept to a minimum. No volume on ethics can provide ready-made answers to the range of moral dilemmas which staff may experience in their work. However, this book does help carers to identify which principles may be relevant in particular situations, and it offers some general guidelines to help staff to decide what actions to take.

Students undertaking National and Scottish Vocational Qualifications (NVQ/SVQ) Care Awards at level 3 should find the book particularly useful, as well as those currently on level 2 and hoping to progress further. The content closely follows the core elements of the Value Base Unit: promoting anti-discriminatory practice; maintaining the confidentiality of information; promoting and supporting an individual's rights; acknowledging an individual's personal beliefs and identity; and supporting individuals through effective communication.

In addition to these areas of competence the text also includes a section on protecting clients from abuse. This is a fundamental unit in a wide variety of NVQ/SVQ courses relevant to the Care Sector Consortium. It is also included because it appears to follow on logically from the content of the previous chapters on values and ethics. Protecting clients from abuse is an area of key concern to care staff and one in which the application of ethical practice is particularly important.

The quality of the environment in residential care accommodation has been improving steadily over the years. More thought has also been given to the need for staff training, as owners and managers of care homes realise the importance of monitoring and raising the standards of care being provided.

The introduction and implementation of National and Scottish Vocational Qualifications in particular have helped in raising the skill levels of care staff, and are continuing to play a significant part in improving standards of practice by stressing the need for good foundation training.

Despite these improvements, there is still concern that cases of abuse in residential and nursing homes continue to occur. Unlike qualified nurses, who are answerable for their conduct to a legally accountable statutory body, there is no similar mechanism to govern the behaviour of other staff employed in the care sector.

Whereas a qualified nurse found guilty of ill-treating clients can be prevented from ever working with vulnerable people again, the same is not true of care assistants or ancillary staff. Even if dismissed for negligent conduct or malpractice, there is nothing to stop them from finding a post with a new, unsuspecting employer. Only if colleagues who witness mistreatment are prepared to speak out and report their misconduct are they likely to be discovered. With this in mind, a chapter on 'whistleblowing' has been included.

The book is intended primarily for the use of student groups on NVQ/SVQ and allied courses. Ethics and values, if they are to be understood properly, require more than a few lectures in a classroom and a quick flick through a couple of text books. Students need to reflect on their own values and those of other people. They also need to listen to the views of others and learn how to debate relevant ethical issues.

To help students consider ethics and values from a practical viewpoint, a number of exercises have been included throughout the text. These can be used by teachers and group leaders to form the basis of student learning activities, either directly or treated as ideas which can be modified. Some of the exercises require students to disclose personal feelings, anxieties and beliefs and not everyone may be enthusiastic to do so at first. However, if students are to increase their understanding of the values which other people hold, they are only likely to achieve this successfully by being prepared to reveal their own.

While it is not necessary to undertake every exercise, to attempt none considerably limits the scope of the book. In some respects, these exercises and the case studies found at the end of each chapter represent the most important part of the book.

A summary of key points is also included at the end of each chapter to serve as a quick reminder of some of the more important issues which have been discussed.

Chapter 1 begins by considering the part that ethics play in everyday life. It goes on to look at values and the key ethical principle of respect for persons and their individual beliefs. Chapter 2 focuses upon the needs of individuals within a group. The conflicts which can arise within a small community and the ethical principles which are relevant to their resolution are discussed.

Chapter 3 looks in some detail at human rights, the different types of rights and the responsibilities that accompany them. Following on from this, Chapter 4 is concerned with effective communication and considers the part that advocacy plays in the client–carer relationship.

The need for care staff to safeguard the privacy of clients, particularly in the area of sexuality, is discussed in Chapter 5. A central theme of this is the importance of maintaining client confidentiality, as well as the reasons that might justify disclosure of confidential information in certain circumstances.

The next three chapters are primarily concerned with abuse and its implications. Chapter 6 deals with the need to promote anti-discriminatory practices in the workplace. Chapter 7 is concerned with protecting clients from abuse and considers what care staff can do to prevent it happening. Chapter 8 concentrates upon the need for staff to report ill treatment when it occurs and the reasons why staff are sometimes reluctant to 'blow the whistle'.

The final chapter discusses how ethics affects the relationships which staff have with each other and with their managers in the working environment.

The book is primarily aimed at those staff who will be, or are, employed in residential care establishments. However, ethics and values are not topics restricted solely to residential and nursing homes. With the arrival of the NHS Community Care Act 1990, more emphasis is now being placed on supporting vulnerable people in their own homes. Care assistants are already involved in providing that support and will continue to do so in the future. An understanding of values and ethics can only improve their knowledge.

Finally, the book assumes that the reader does not have detailed knowledge of ethics – only a willingness to learn.

Chapter 1
Respect for Persons

Ethics and the principle of respect

Respect for persons is an ethical principle of paramount importance to care workers. It is essential for establishing relationships with clients and with other people we meet. It involves, among other things, being truthful and keeping promises. Without it, life would be chaotic.

Imagine, for instance, being reassured by a porter that a certain train was travelling to Newcastle, only to discover later, as the train entered Plymouth, that he had been lying! Or imagine buying a washing machine and the following week a new refrigerator is delivered instead. Whether purchasing goods from a shop, attending a GP's surgery or sitting as a student in class, the success of our daily activities depends on people telling us the truth. Besides making life more orderly, telling the truth demonstrates respect for people and a concern for their feelings.

Respect has become something of an old fashioned word, perhaps because in the past it has been linked too often with authority or power. Children in particular have been urged to respect their 'betters', meaning people in positions of power, or to show respect to institutions such as the law or the established church. But the ethical principle of respect for persons stands for something different. It signifies that we should never treat people merely as a means to an end.

It would be wrong, for instance, to use individuals for scientific experiments who were unable to give consent. Treating people as guinea pigs merely to advance scientific knowledge does not show respect for them as human beings. Ways have to be found for research to take place in a manner which respects those subjects taking part.

Similarly, the need for hygiene in a residential home is important to keep potential infections at bay. It would be wrong, however, to treat the bathing of clients simply as a means to achieve the end of a clean environment. We may clean our car with one end in mind – to make it look shiny and bright – but people need to be treated differently. People require privacy. Few individuals would enjoy being left naked before the bath and exposed to public view. How someone is bathed is as important as the final state of cleanliness they achieve. Hygiene is not even the only reason why people like to bathe. A warm bath is comforting to wallow in and some clients may want a bath simply to relax. Showing respect for the individual needs of clients is demonstrating respect for them as people.

Ethics are a branch of philosophy that focuses on matters of right and wrong, or good and bad. They tell people how they *ought* to treat each other. Ethics also state that individuals are of equal value, which means that if lying is wrong, it is wrong for everybody. A manager who expects his or her staff to be truthful has to abide by the same rules. The same holds true for making promises.

Ethics recognise that there are degrees of good and bad. The type of promise and the circumstances involved in making it are important. A promise to love, cherish and obey a spouse is more solemn than one to return a book to a friend. Intentions play a significant part in ethics, and being unable to keep a promise is more forgivable than making one but having no intention of keeping it.

Demonstrating respect for individuals relates to the ethical principle of veracity (or truth telling and keeping promises). Other principles, which will be discussed in later chapters, are also involved. For now, it is enough to say that ethical principles apply equally to everyone, to both staff and clients alike.

 Action exercise 1.1 _____

Give reasons why some promises are broken and discuss circumstances which could possibly justify breaking a promise.

Failure to respect persons

Being an individual, or a person, is something we spend comparatively little time thinking about: we take it for granted. Sometimes however, it is necessary to consider whether a human being still retains the characteristics of personhood.

The question can arise when relatives of someone in a deep coma request doctors to switch off the machinery keeping the patient alive. To them, the body lying connected to the life-support machine is no longer a person in the generally accepted sense, especially if the coma is likely to be irreversible.

Care workers are not normally likely to participate in tragic circumstances such as these. Nevertheless, understanding about respect for persons is important to ethical practice. It can be extremely difficult sometimes to define exactly whether a living organism is actually a person. These uncertainties are often at the heart of controversial ethical debates. Opinions on abortion, for example, vary according to whether a person considers a foetus to be a human being, or merely a collection of cells with the potential to develop into one.

Philosophers often try to identify features that are uniquely human. Nearly all agree that characteristics like consciousness and self-awareness are vital. Some feel that an ability to relate or communicate with other people is essential, while still others argue that a sense of curiosity and the ability to adapt to a changing environment are fundamental necessities for a living being to be considered human.

A few clients living in residential homes are unlikely to match all of the so-called characteristics which philosophers cite. Some clients, because of confusion, may not always be aware of their surroundings while others may appear to lack an ability to relate meaningfully to other individuals. In the case of some clients, apathy may stifle natural curiosity.

Appearances, however, can be deceptive. Regardless of any characteristics which may be lacking, clients should always have their individuality respected. In the past, clients living in institutions have been described in appalling ways. Staff have even referred to some as 'cabbages' or 'vegetables'. Predictably, this failure to respect people as human beings has led to inhumane treatment.

Treating people without respect invariably means treating them badly. Even well-intentioned members of the public can be guilty of hurtful thoughtlessness. They often treat people with special needs as being invisible, ignoring them by not asking them things directly but addressing questions instead to the person by their side. If asked why they act this way, people will explain that they did not realise that the handicapped person could respond to the question. However, this does not prevent many from going home and talking to their household pets. Deliberately ignoring an individual is an insult, not a mark of respect, regardless of whether the person rejected realises it or not.

There have been cases of hospital patients in a seemingly permanent coma who have made unexpected recoveries. Some have recalled how they could hear and understand what people around them were saying, even though they themselves could not communicate with the world. Hearing is often the last of the senses to be lost and patients have recounted snatches of conversations overheard from medical and nursing staff with sometimes less than kind remarks made about themselves.

This underlines the importance of treating people with respect, whether or not they appear to be conscious of their surroundings. It is a mistake to think that an elderly person who suffers from dementia or a young person with a severe learning disability is never capable of understanding what is said to them. Only by treating individuals as humans can we be sure of treating them humanely.

Identity and forms of address

Although people share much in common they also have many differences. Just as they vary in appearance, they also do in other factors. The effects of environment, genetic inheritance and personal beliefs play a crucial part in the development of identity. Brothers and sisters may look alike and share a common family upbringing but they have their own unique differences. These contrasts serve to remind people that instead of being mere mirror images of each other they are individuals with a unique personality of their own.

Many factors go to make up our personality, including physical and mental attributes, such as powers of concentration and intelligence. Our temperament, whether placid and patient or fiery and impulsive, also shapes the ways in which we express our inner selves. Our attitudes, beliefs, interests and future hopes are other characteristics we present to the world in the form of personal identity. While we may not like every aspect of our personality, we cherish it as being the outward mark of our own unique self.

A person's name is one of the more obvious characteristics of their identity. People enjoy being recognised which is why they feel awkward if they forget the name or face of an acquaintance they meet. Addressing someone by name gives recognition to their individuality and singles them out from the crowd.

Names are so important that if an individual dislikes the ones given at birth they may choose different ones in later life. Even in marriage, a woman does not have to take her husband's surname. For a variety of reasons she may want to keep her own. Some couples even choose to start married life with a new, joint, hyphenated name comprising both their former surnames.

Formal names are not to everyone's liking. Some prefer instead to use a nickname or a pet name, only revealing their real name if they have to sign legal documents. Quite often the names that appear in a client's notes might not be the one that he or she prefers to use. One of the first things that care staff should do, when a client is newly admitted to a residential home, is discover what name the client prefers, and how they like to be addressed. This can vary according to circumstances. An elderly lady chatting to fellow residents may be quite happy to be called 'Maisie' by her peers. However, when addressed by a young member of staff she may prefer being called 'Mrs Jones'.

Displaying respect for people means addressing them in the manner they prefer and being sensitive to their needs. Asking for a client's Christian name, instead of his or her first name, can be offensive if that person is a non-believer or practises a non-Christian religion.

People's names and personalities reflect their individuality. Just as care staff wish to express their own individuality in their own way the same holds true for their clients.

 Action exercise 1.2

Write a brief description of your own personality as you perceive it, including those aspects that you like the most and those which you would most like to change.
Write a brief description of a partner's personality as you see it. Exchange the written descriptions with each other to see how closely

they match. Discuss your perceptions and the relative strengths and weaknesses identified.

Beliefs

The beliefs that we hold are an important part of our identity. Whether they are religious, cultural or moral beliefs, they are precious because they reflect who we are and how we live our lives; they influence both our behaviour and our needs.

For example, individuals with strong spiritual beliefs will almost certainly want to attend religious services with fellow worshippers. Similarly those who on grounds of principle choose not to eat meat need a vegetarian menu.

Most people living in democratic countries experience comparatively little difficulty in practising their beliefs. Circumstances can and do change, however. Growing old can cause a decline in the ability to undertake the normal activities of life. Individuals who once were able to make their own way to church may come to rely upon others to take them. When clients experience a loss of independence this places a greater burden upon staff, for as well as encouraging residents to express their wishes and beliefs, staff also have to help clients practise them.

Beliefs exert a powerful hold on human behaviour, sometimes in a negative way. Individuals can be fooled at times by false beliefs. A client suffering from paranoia could believe that staff were poisoning his or her food and consequently refuse to eat it.

In some cases beliefs can motivate people to spend substantial amounts of time engaging in particular activities. Often people seek out others who share the same convictions to create organisations that reflect their mutual viewpoints. Political bodies, such as animal rights organisations and environmental groups, owe their existence to the individual beliefs of their members.

The number and range of beliefs that human beings hold are incredibly diverse. Individuals can harbour strong convictions about the way they dress, their attitudes towards illness or how they spend their money. What is important to one person may be insignificant to someone else. Beliefs do not necessarily have to be true in order to influence behaviour. Comparatively few people join the 'flat earth society' or believe in flying saucers. Nevertheless those who do hold these convictions spend time in pursuing these interests and in discussion with fellow believers.

Conflicts between beliefs

Care workers will not necessarily share the same beliefs as the clients they look after. Normally this should not be a problem, but inevitably there will be times when there is a direct conflict between the beliefs of a client and those of a carer. In social situations outside the workplace, it is possible for people to avoid those with whom they violently disagree. Alternatively, they can set out to convert others to their way of thinking. These options, however, are not open to carers when they are on duty and interacting with their clients. It is best for staff who disagree with the beliefs of their clients, to maintain a tactful silence and not allow themselves to be drawn into arguments.

Part of a carer's role is to promote the rights of the people they are looking after. Clients have a right to freedom of speech and therefore to express their opinions, regardless of their carer's viewpoints, providing this does not cause harm to others.

Despite this, some clients may feel reluctant to express their opinions, if they believe that they are in conflict with those of the staff. The reason for this is that the relationship between clients and carers is an unequal one. An imbalance of power exists between the two, particularly for the more dependent clients.

Staff have to meet the needs of a number of individuals, and because they cannot attend to everyone at the same time they must prioritise their duties. Some clients wanting assistance with bathing, for instance, will have to wait for a carer to be free from other tasks. Less able clients, therefore, are reliant upon the priorities of the workforce. In comparison to individuals who need less help, they may not want to upset staff, and consequently may find it more difficult to speak their minds, especially if their opinions contrast strongly with those of their carers. Alternatively, they may pretend to agree with their carer's viewpoint simply 'for a quiet life'.

Clients who are dependent on others have little control over their environment. Consequently, they can become resigned to the daily routine, submitting passively to it and never questioning any aspect of it. The problem for staff is how to minimise the inequalities that exist, while at the same time dispensing care in an effective manner. The potential one-sidedness of the client–carer relationship poses a challenge for staff who have the task of trying to make it a more equal one.

Values

Values are a particular type of belief concerned with the worth of an idea or type of behaviour. They represent standards that influence many of the judgements that we make. They also relate to the ways in which we look at ourselves and at the world at large. Like other aspects of our belief system, values arise from a number of different sources.

Parents and other significant adults are mainly responsible for the values we adopt as children. As we grow older, friends, peers, and other powerful role models contribute to our developing value system. Life events and the lessons learned from them can also strongly influence the values we hold.

In addition to personal values, there are also cultural ones which are often shared by members of the same community or background. People from different communities, however, may possess similar values often because of common experiences.

During the Second World War, both the British and the German civilian population experienced rationing and food shortages. People living through that period may value thrift and detest unnecessary wastage more than those born in comparatively affluent times. Indeed, younger generations may not value thrift at all. To them it may be too closely associated with miserly characteristics and selfishness. Instead they may value the widespread distribution of resources for everyone's benefit today, without too much concern for what will happen tomorrow. This is not to say that all older people value thrift or that all younger persons do not, it is only an example of how a common experience may influence people to adopt a particular value.

Unlike some beliefs, values are not necessarily right or wrong.

While it is possible to prove correct a belief that the world is round, values cannot be similarly tested. Valuing thrift is no more 'correct' or 'right' than valuing generosity.

Values can change in the same way that a person's circumstances can. Many people may not particularly value their job, but if they were suddenly to be told they were to be made redundant, their employment may seem more precious to them. Another example is when a relationship has broken up, and one or more of the partners looks back and realise that something worthwhile has been lost.

Some values remain with individuals throughout their lives. Academic people often retain a life-long interest in learning, long after they have passed all the exams necessary to enhance their careers. This is because they value the pursuit of knowledge for its own sake.

The values held by people with contrasting lifestyles will often be different. It is not surprising, therefore, that lifestyles of client and carer will sometimes vary. What is important is that people do not try to impose their values upon other individuals. Care workers in particular should respect the values of their clients, whether or not they share them.

Action exercise 1.3

Identify characteristics that you value and others that you do not, in someone who is a close friend. Repeat the exercise for someone who is not a friend but might be influential in your life (a teacher, employer, etc.). Compare lists with other group members to discuss what effect characteristics (both valued and not valued) might have on different types of relationship.

Behaviour

The relationship between beliefs and behaviour is a close one. Ignoring the beliefs of an individual, or acting in opposition to them, can have an adverse effect on their behaviour. For instance, clients who believe alcohol is a vice are unlikely to welcome a visit to a pub. Similarly, if a resident believes that domestic pets are unhygienic, they are likely to protest loudly if they find one sleeping on their bed.

Both beliefs and behaviours are subject to change as people grow older. Young children often show an unquestioning acceptance of the authority of parents and teachers. But as they grow older, the realisation dawns that adults, like children, can make mistakes. During adolescence teenagers modify many existing beliefs and establish new ones. Far from being seen as sources of wisdom, they often see the older generation as being old-fashioned and out of date.

Some young people adopt intense beliefs in political causes and join protest movements to demonstrate their support for their new found interests, others prefer to devote themselves to living for the moment and enjoying the company of new friends. On entering adulthood, behaviour and beliefs often change again. Many individuals take on increased responsibilities by setting up home with a partner or starting a new family. Consequently, their domestic life often takes precedence over their social activities as they settle into new relationships.

With advancing years, people's beliefs and behaviour continue to change. The energies of youth are reduced. They may become less physically active and enthusiastic about tackling new projects. Sometimes these changes are accompanied by a philosophical outlook which is more accepting of life's limitations.

Life crises can have a dramatic effect upon both beliefs and behaviour. Traumatic events such as unemployment, family break-up, serious illness, or bereavement can sometimes lead people to modify or abandon formerly strongly held beliefs. However, not everyone reacts in the same way, even when their circumstances are similar.

For some individuals, divorce may leave them with feelings of great bitterness, as well as a determination never again to place their trust in another human being. Other individuals may see it as an opportunity to make a fresh start and seek out a more compatible partner.

In a similar way clients can show very different reactions when moving into a residential care home. Some may be bitter, feeling that their family have abandoned them. They can exhibit over-critical behaviour of their new surroundings and of the people who work within it. Others, pleased not to become a burden on their children, may welcome the move into a new environment and be grateful for the help that is on offer. Staff should be aware that the behaviour they see when someone is first admitted may not be typical of what an individual usually displays. Some residents will need more support and understanding than others at such times.

Conscience

Forcing anyone to act against their beliefs is wrong. This is why some ethical codes of conduct contain 'conscience clauses' allowing staff to refrain from taking part in activities which they think are wrong. For example, nurses in the UK who take the view that abortion is wrong, do not have to assist in operations involving the termination of pregnancies. People who hold strong feelings that war is wrong are similarly allowed to refrain from joining the fighting services, if they meet the criteria to be classed as a conscientious objector.

Conscience is a set of beliefs that is capable of invoking powerful emotional feelings within an individual. Most people, at some time or other, experience guilt or regret about things they have done, or failed to do. Many feel distress if they ignore their conscience or are prevented from exercising it. It is therefore useful if staff are aware of any strong moral convictions which their clients hold, if only to avoid unintentional offence.

Although conscience can have an ethical dimension it is not always the best guide to ethical behaviour. If it was that simple, people would only have to act according to their consciences and not bother about ethics. Individuals, however, can be mistaken in holding strong convictions.

A deprived child growing up in an environment where crime is the norm, might see nothing wrong in stealing from those they consider to be rich, particularly if they have been presented with poor role models by parents or siblings. Yet stealing is wrong regardless of the circumstances, and crime does not become acceptable because someone is not conscience-stricken when committing it.

A mother in extreme poverty might steal food for her children. To see them go hungry could stir her conscience to such an extent that she felt she had no alternative but to go shoplifting. Many people would feel sympathy for someone in her circumstances and be prepared to make allowances for her if she was caught in the act. Yet, stealing from others is nevertheless a crime, regardless of whether or not an individual is punished for it. Once a person decides it is justifiable for them to break the law there is nothing to prevent others from doing the same.

During the Second World War, Hitler's conscience was not troubled by his treatment of Jews or of mentally ill people, thousands of whom were ultimately exterminated. Although individuals like Hitler are thankfully rare, many normal people can be misled by false perceptions of conscience.

Sometimes people feel guilty even when they have done nothing wrong, particularly when a person they love dies. Similarly, individuals sometimes feel guilty, despite devoting years to looking after a loved one, if they can no longer cope and they have to relinquish their role to paid carers.

Just as conscience can be mistaken in making people feel guilty, it can also be unreliable in telling them when they are at fault. Forgetfulness can silence conscience, as when a memory lapse prevents us from remembering a promise we have made.

Care workers should respect the consciences of clients and other carers too. Although acting according to conscience does not always guarantee ethical behaviour, it is often unethical to make someone deliberately act against their conscience.

Autonomy

People cherish the freedom to express their beliefs, to make their own decisions and to be in control of their own destiny. The name we give that freedom is autonomy and it is one of the most valued aspects of personhood. If for any reason people are deprived of their autonomy, then their sense of individuality can be diminished. Inevitably, many of the clients that we care for will experience a loss of autonomy. Merely being dependent upon a carer for help in dressing, eating, or bathing, reduces the amount of control that a client has over his or her own destiny.

Nobody, of course, has complete freedom all the time. As employees, people have to attend work on a regular basis and obey the boss's orders. In theory they are at liberty to leave their jobs.

However, because the rent or mortgage needs paying the freedom is more illusory than real.

Other factors can also restrict our autonomy. If two shoppers both decide that they would like to buy a particular dress in a sale, one of them is going to be disappointed, if it is the only garment of its type remaining. We tend to accept these comparatively petty constraints placed on our personal liberty as a reasonable price to pay for living in a free society where, in the main, we can exert significant control over our own lives.

The loss of control which clients experience, because of their dependency, places a responsibility upon carers to find ways to increase client autonomy whenever possible. If clients have to be dressed by staff, it becomes even more important that they select the clothes they want to wear. Similarly, residents who are unable to bathe themselves may still be capable of making choices. Staff can find out whether clients would rather have a shower instead of a bath. The preferences of clients should be respected whenever possible. Some individuals prefer an early morning shower while others would rather have a leisurely soak in the evening. Involving clients in decision making helps to empower them and provides them with a measure of autonomy.

If staff make too many decisions on behalf of clients, they can induce in them a state of learned helplessness. Clients in this condition lose the will to interest themselves in originating any activities. Instead, they become passive recipients of care with their autonomy reduced even further.

As well as helping clients to make decisions, staff can encourage them to express their opinions and speak about their interests. Good communication skills, which include the ability to listen actively and make appropriate responses, are an essential part of a care-worker's skills.

Most people positively welcome the opportunity to express their own opinions, but a few clients may value their privacy too much to reveal many things about themselves. Individuals are entitled to their privacy. If they are reluctant to talk about themselves, staff can help them by respecting their reticence and not intrude unnecessarily.

Client records

Client records usually contain information that can be useful in building up a picture of an individual and obtaining an insight into their personal preferences. However, caution has to be exercised in relying too much upon them too soon in a relationship. It is always preferable to get to know a client by personal interaction first, before reading someone else's notes about them.

Unfortunately written records are not always accurate, and, in the case of hand-written ones, not always legible. Even when information is both clear and correct, some of the notes about an individual can be biased. Sometimes, comparatively minor incidents are magnified out of all proportion. A sudden fit of frustration that leads a client to throw an object across a room can label a client as 'having aggressive tendencies', even though it might have been an isolated incident.

Reading such a description, new staff not knowing the clients very well might think that they are dealing with a potentially violent person. This can result in them adopting an unnecessarily defensive attitude towards a client that is detrimental to any future relationship.

Most of us at some time or other have been guilty of isolated incidents of behaviour that we would prefer to forget. We would doubtless be horrified, if told that an action, of which we were not particularly proud, had been recorded permanently on a document to which many people had access.

Careful thought has to be given before making entries into personal records. Once a comment is entered into a record it tends to remain there unaltered. Respecting people means treating them fairly and honestly. If an individual does display regular episodes of aggressive behaviour then it makes sense to report the incidents. If it is a single act of aggression, it should be pointed out that the behaviour is untypical and out of character.

 Action exercise 1.4 _____

Write a brief concise description (no more than one side of an A4 size piece of paper) of an event or place that all members of the group have witnessed (i.e. a television programme or a visit to a particular place).

Exchange your description with one written by another group member and out of a maximum of ten points mark it according to how well you judge it to be written. Such things as accuracy, clarity, amount of relevant detail or quality of objective reporting might be some of the things for which you are looking. Descriptions are circulated among the group members who all allocate marks. Total the marks and rank descriptions according to their score. Group members then discuss whether they agree with the overall ranking or not.

It is important to record both consistent and inconsistent patterns of behaviour. It is in the client's best interests to do so. Unusual or irregular behaviour can sometimes signal the onset of serious illness or a deterioration in functioning, which medical, psychological or therapeutic interventions might be able to ease. When writing information in client records it is vital to do it clearly, concisely, and without prejudice.

In addition to recording information it is also essential to check it for accuracy. Any mistakes or discrepancies that find their way into records should be reported to senior staff. If carers are uncertain whether something should be recorded or not they should refer to senior staff for advice. The aim is to produce a document that reflects information truthfully in an unbiased way.

A point that will be made throughout this book is that if care-workers experience *any* problems relating to particular clients, they should seek the support and guidance of senior staff. When caring for vulnerable people, a major ethical principle is to always strive to act in their best interests.

There will be times when carers are uncertain as to what represents the best interests of a client, especially when they are new to the job. To discount the possibility of more experienced staff being able to identify what is best for the individual, by not seeking their support, is to needlessly jeopardise the well-being of clients.

 Case study _____

Mrs Holder is an 80 year old lady confined to a wheelchair. She has strong religious beliefs and is taken by a member of staff every Sunday to the local church that is about a mile away. Recently she has been requesting to be taken to additional services in the week. She has no visitors and if a member of staff takes her this will seriously reduce the number of staff available to attend to the needs of other residents. Discuss how this situation might be handled.

Summary of key points

- Respect for persons is a key ethical principle.
- Ethics are concerned with right and wrong and guide us in how we *ought* to respect and treat each other as individuals.
- Ethics are the foundation stone upon which the concept of equality for all individuals is based.
- Individuals need to express their personal identity and value being addressed in a preferred manner.
- Clients should be encouraged to declare their beliefs providing they are not harmful to other people.
- Beliefs affect behaviour and if people are prevented from expressing their convictions it can adversely affect their conduct.
- A power imbalance exists in the relationship between client and carer which can inhibit clients from stating their true beliefs.
- As people mature and develop their beliefs and behaviours are subject to change.
- Individuals value autonomy which is the freedom to control and make decisions concerning how they live.
- Care workers require good communication skills to encourage clients to discuss their needs.

Chapter 2
The Individual within the Group

Needs and quality of life

Everybody has needs that have to be met in order to live. Needs that are common to everyone are those that are essential for life, like food, air, water, sleep, warmth and security. Closely following these basic requirements are other important ones, if life is to be something more than mere survival.

Most people, for instance, have a need to give and receive affection. They also have a desire to feel good about themselves. Feelings of low self-esteem or a lack of emotional warmth tend to suppress an individual's capacity for happiness.

Despite people having many needs in common, they also have others which are very different. A professional footballer must be fully fit to be selected for his club team. His livelihood and that of his family depend to a great degree upon him avoiding injuries. By contrast, a minor physical injury is relatively unimportant to a philosopher. Instead, he or she requires an academic environment that provides a stimulating, but non-disruptive, atmosphere in which to think and concentrate.

The needs of people living within a residential home reflect those of the people living outside it. To some extent, personal likes and dislikes will influence the needs of clients. Those who are artistic for instance, may see painting or needlework as an essential part of a happy life whereas someone totally uninterested in art will not be concerned if it is missing from their lives.

The degree to which individuals are able to satisfy their desires is crucial to the quality of their life. People who feel that their life has little or no quality, as well as being unhappy, often lose the will to live. The major argument in favour of euthanasia rests upon the idea that it is better to be dead, than living a life of misery. Consequently, people in great pain, or suffering from an incurable disease, sometimes plead with doctors to end their misery.

In this country it is still illegal for doctors, or anyone else, to help people to take their own life. Thankfully, staff working in care homes are not likely to come across clients in such extreme circumstances in their daily practice. However, it is necessary for staff to appreciate how the satisfaction of personal needs relates to clients maintaining an acceptable quality of life.

It is not only physical pain that can drive some people to contemplate taking drastic remedies to obtain relief. In some cases it is because many of the needs that are important to them can no longer be fulfilled. Everybody's job is important to them, but for some it occupies nearly their whole life. It provides them not only with the means to live, but with status and interest which fulfils many of their personal ambitions. For them redundancy can be especially shattering and their quality of life irrevocably damaged.

Similarly, the mental anguish caused by breakdowns in a close relationship is something which many people experience. But for some, the realisation that they are no longer wanted as before becomes almost impossible to bear and they sink into depression, not caring if they live or die.

It is usually possible for individuals to come to terms with the fact that some of their needs will remain unfulfilled. The extent to which personal desires affect different individuals varies tremendously, and the influence they have on a person's quality of life cannot be underestimated. Care staff have a duty to help clients experience a good quality of life, which means assisting them to satisfy as many of their needs as possible.

Translocation shock

Stability is a need common to many people. Sudden and abrupt changes of lifestyle can produce stresses that result in devastating effects upon an individual's health. Admission to a residential home can be an extremely traumatic experience, particularly for an elderly person who has had to leave the familiar environment of their home after many years. A client with learning difficulties, who leaves a large long-stay institution to live in a home in the community, is similarly vulnerable to the stresses of sudden change.

Care staff should be aware of these dangers. Research studies by psychologists have identified some of the traumas that can arise from translocation shock, or relocation syndrome, as it is also known. These can range from behavioural disturbances to physical illnesses, depression and, in rare circumstances, death.

Careful planning should take place before admission. Ideally, this should involve a gradual introduction to the new and unfamiliar surroundings. However, emergencies do arise and sometimes clients are admitted at short notice. The need to establish roots in the new environment is crucial, and it is important for staff to help clients settle in and set up fresh routines.

It is possible to minimise the potential danger of translocation shock. Helping clients to maintain links with their previous life is one positive step. This can be done by encouraging them to bring in photographs of significant people and personal mementoes. Visits by relatives and former friends are also helpful. If it is possible for clients to continue with interests and hobbies they previously enjoyed, they should be encouraged to do so. At this stage in a client's life they are particularly vulnerable, and their requirements for security, reassurance and new routines are especially important.

Fulfilment of needs

Carers, by their actions in the work setting, must ensure that their client's needs receive equal recognition. This does not mean that all clients will receive identical care or treatment. Some clients will have requirements that are more demanding than others. Someone who is incapable of feeding him or herself, for example, will require more assistance than a person who is completely independent.

A few individuals may have requirements that are impossible to satisfy. Although incapable of looking after themselves, some clients may want to return to their own homes. Unfortunately, if their families are unable to cope with caring for them, there is little chance of them being able to do so.

Recognition of needs means that staff should recognise that all of the requirements of a client are important. Even if a client expresses a need that appears to be superficial, it is not the carer's role to downgrade the significance of it. What is important to one individual may be considered trivial by another.

Respecting the needs of clients means more than just taking them seriously. If it is impossible to meet a particular requirement, care staff must explain the reasons why. Furthermore, every effort should be made to fulfil complementary needs. A client who wants to return home but is unable to do so, has other related needs to consider. Moving away from home inevitably means that the client experiences a substantial loss of contact with his or her family. A client's related need for increased contact with relatives could be partially satisfied if staff could persuade the family to visit more often, or arrange extra weekend breaks at home.

Equal recognition of needs means considering the requirements of all clients. However, there can be occasions when it is justifiable to prevent an individual from fulfilling a personal need, if satisfying it adversely affects other people.

 Action exercise 2.1 _____

Compile a written list of needs that must be met for most people to enjoy a reasonable quality of life. Compare your list with other group members to find which needs are common and which are not. Discuss possible reasons to account for any differences.

When needs conflict

People do not exist solely as individuals, they also belong to groups. Consequently the needs they have can sometimes conflict with those of other group members. The first group that people belong to is the family. It is usually also where they experience their first conflicts. Later as individuals grow and develop, they become members of an increasing number of other groups, at school, college, work and in their social life.

Whenever a group forms, there is always a potential for conflict amongst its members. Most of us will have had some experience, no matter how minor, of conflicts between friends at school or colleagues at work. Clients, as well as being individuals in their own right, are also members of a shared community of residents. Inevitably there will be times when conflicts arise because the needs of individuals within the community clash.

When friction results because of conflicts, it is often the care-worker who has to try to resolve the situation. Care staff have a duty to attend to the needs of all clients in their care, not those of just one individual, however likeable or important that person might be.

Situations can arise in communal living when the behaviour of one person can upset the remaining members of the group. For example, most people require an undisturbed night's sleep of seven or eight hours. A few individuals can do with considerably less. If a particular client only requires three or four hours' sleep and on waking decides to wander around the premises, then other residents are going to protest. Nobody enjoys having a disturbed night's sleep.

Unfortunately, it is not always possible to resolve conflicts among clients to everybody's satisfaction. In this case, whatever course of action a member of staff takes, it will almost certainly result in someone feeling aggrieved. To allow the wanderer to continue roaming promotes his or her autonomy, but causes strife to almost everyone else, whereas preventing the client from engaging in a nightly walkabout pleases everybody else, but restricts the client's personal freedom.

Sometimes it is possible to resolve conflicts through compromise. In an establishment where residents all have private accommodation, it is easier to persuade clients who wake early to remain in their rooms, to avoid disturbing other people. Compromises, however, are not always so conveniently available. Occasions will arise when the needs of one or more individuals have to be overridden, because they clash with those of other group members. The dilemma facing care staff is to determine which needs, if any, have priority, and how to justify decisions that prevent some clients from expressing their autonomy.

Harm to self and others

A powerful justification for preventing an individual from satisfying a personal need is if, in doing so, it causes a substantial amount of harm. In Chapter 1, we saw that carers should respect and encourage the beliefs and wishes of an individual, providing that they do not result in harm either to the individual concerned or to other people.

In any relationship where one person is dependent upon another a duty of care exists. In the relationship between carer and client, a prime duty of the staff is to safeguard the interests of clients by protecting them from harm. Qualified nurses are answerable to the Code of Professional Conduct, which states that nurses should always act in a patient's best interests. Likewise, doctors are taught in their ethical codes of practice that, above everything else, patients must be protected from harm.

This fundamental ethical rule applies as much to direct care staff as it does to any other professionals working in the field of health or social care. Clients entrusted to our care should not be worse off as a result. Some clients will suffer from confusion or depression. Because of this, the wishes they express, or the beliefs they cling to, may not always be in their own best interests.

Those with a mental illness can sometimes become deluded and even believe that staff are trying to poison them. Consequently, they may refuse to eat their food. In circumstances like these care workers will have to act; they cannot allow clients to recklessly endanger their lives. At the very least, they will have to report the situation to a senior member of staff.

It is impossible to protect clients from all sources of harm. Sometimes it is necessary to tolerate a small amount of harm to prevent a more serious one. When people fall ill, they may require drugs to be injected into them. Although few individuals welcome the sight of a syringe, most people willingly tolerate the minor pin prick of an injection, in exchange for relief from discomfort or pain.

In helping clients to maintain a reasonable quality of life, staff can find themselves in an ethical dilemma. Somehow they have to strike a balance between protecting individuals from harm and allowing them to take acceptable risks. The nature and severity of potential risks have to be assessed. An elderly gentleman who is unsteady on his feet may refuse the assistance of a helping arm as he makes his way across the day room. Respecting his feelings of independence staff may stand nearby but refrain from helping him. If the same gentleman expressed a similar desire to cross a busy main road however, it would be irresponsible to allow him to attempt to do so. It is because staff have a duty to protect clients from harm that there may be occasions when, in the interests of safety, they have to overrule the wishes of a client.

So important is the duty to avoid harm, that many policies and controls have been designed for the protection of people at risk. In the working environment these range from fire regulations to procedures regarding manual lifting. Employers in the public, private and voluntary organisations, as well as the individuals who work for them, also have duties of care.

Legislation such as the Health and Safety at Work Act 1974 and the Food Safety Act 1990, exists for the protection of the public. Promoting public safety inevitably imposes some restrictions on personal freedom. Even if employees are prepared to take personal risks at work, the law does not allow them to put themselves or others in danger. Similarly, care staff sometimes have to act paternalistically and overrule decisions made by clients that could be detrimental to the safety of themselves or others.

 Action exercise 2.2

Search out details of any other regulations, legislation or organisations that exist to protect people from harm. Also, find any policies or procedures that are designed to safeguard clients in care establishments.

Paternalism

The word paternalism literally means 'government as by a father'. When carers act paternalistically they are doing so in the same way that a parent does when making decisions on behalf of a child. Normally clients want to make their own decisions, and the last thing they want is for care staff to treat them like children.

However, respect for persons means having a concern for their welfare, as well as a regard for their wishes. The welfare of clients takes priority over a regard for their wishes, if the choices they make risk causing them serious harm. For example, a youngster with learning difficulties, reaching puberty and conscious perhaps for the first time of strong sexual feelings, may feel an urge to undress and expose him or herself to public view.

This type of behaviour clearly carries with it a serious risk of harm. Firstly, it makes the individual vulnerable to unscrupulous people who might exploit them sexually, and secondly, it puts them in breach of the law and at risk of prosecution. In addition, it is behaviour that conflicts with the needs of others, who may feel embarrassed or even disgusted at the spectacle. In a case like this, carers have a duty to overrule the youngster's autonomy and act paternalistically. They cannot allow clients to engage in illegal activities, even if it means in the short-term that a member of staff must always escort them when they are out.

When staff have to prevent clients from taking unwise decisions, it is important that they do so in a proper manner. Overruling a client's autonomy is an unfortunate necessity, and to do it in a way that belittles an individual is unacceptable. Adults should be treated appropriately for their age, and if certain behaviour cannot be allowed, staff must explain respectfully the reasons why.

Explanations should never be withheld, even if it is uncertain how much a client understands. Otherwise, it is all too easy for staff to fall into the habit of not bothering to explain. Even when clients do not understand explanations, the tone of voice used can reassure them that the carer is not angry with them.

When staff do have to curb a client's behaviour, it becomes even more necessary to find ways to promote their autonomy in the future. A client who expresses his or her sexuality in an unsuitable way is probably unaware of the most appropriate way of doing so. Merely prohibiting a client's behaviour is not enough. Carers have to strike a balance between taking paternalistic action designed to prohibit antisocial behaviour and making plans to promote the future autonomy of the client. This can be done by teaching the client to display more socially acceptable behaviour and to learn new skills.

Utilitarianism – the theory of utility

It is justifiable to restrict the behaviour of an individual if it threatens the well-being of other members of a group. In ethics there is a theory that takes this reasoning even further. It goes under the rather daunting name of utilitarianism, or the theory of utility.

Put simply, the theory measures the 'rightness' of an action by calculating the number of people who benefit by it. Someone who believes in the theory is known as a utilitarian. He or she will try to resolve ethical dilemmas by deciding which actions give the greatest value to the majority of people. In the case of the restless client disturbing others at night, a utilitarian would restrict the movements of the wanderer. This would allow the greatest number of people to benefit by enjoying a decent night's sleep.

The theory is more popularly known 'as doing the greatest good for the greatest number'. In some circumstances it is not possible to bring about much in the way of good, for example, when a fire breaks out in a building. In these situations, the aim of a utilitarian is to see that most people come to as little harm as possible.

One of the disadvantages of utilitarianism is that it often disregards minority interests. Consequently there is a risk that some individuals will always lose out. Imagine, for instance, a situation where only seven clients, from a total of twenty, can go on a weekly minibus trip. The reasons why so few can go are not important. It could be due to lack of staff, availability of transport, or for some other reason. Ideally, seven different clients should go each week, until all those who want an outing have had one. However, what if two clients regularly exhibit challenging behaviours? These could take the form of verbal or physical aggression or other antisocial acts. Not only will these disruptions probably upset other passengers, they are also likely to demand more staff attention. Consequently, less will be available for the rest of the party. Almost certainly both staff and clients will have a much more peaceful time if the 'unruly' individuals are left behind.

Taking a utilitarian approach, excluding the clients with challenging behaviours from social outings undoubtedly benefits the most people, but the cost of this benefit is much too high. Excluding 'socially disruptive' individuals from activities is effectively punishing them for behaviour over which they may have little or no control.

Justifying exclusions

Penalising an innocent person for the benefit of others is not ethically justifiable. Including clients with challenging behaviours in group activities makes extra work for staff. Other residents may also find their behaviour discomforting. However, neither minor discomforts nor an additional workload are adequate reasons to justify preventing so-called disruptive individuals from joining in group activities.

Staff must treat all clients fairly. To do this, it is sometimes necessary to search for alternative solutions to difficult problems. In this case, when clients requiring extra attention are included in the party, the answer could be to reduce the total number of clients on the minibus.

There can be occasions when it is justifiable to take a utilitarian approach, especially if it protects many people from a risk of *substantial* harm. A client with a highly infectious condition should be isolated from others, to avoid spreading it to them. Once the condition improves however, staff should encourage the individual to resume his or her usual activities.

There are many different types of utilitarianism and the welfare state is largely the result of thinkers who were strong advocates of the philosophy. There is much to be said in its favour. Nevertheless, it carries with it the danger of failing to protect minority interests.

At times, staff will find it necessary to take decisions for the benefit of the majority of clients. This is acceptable practice, providing that each situation is looked at according to its merits. Staff have a duty to serve the interests of all clients.

Care staff, especially those new to the job, are not expected to make paternalistic decisions on their own. They lack the experience to do so and they may be too much under the influence of their own beliefs and upbringing. Personal prejudices affect us all and care staff are no different from anyone else. The values they hold influence the way that they behave.

People come from a variety of different backgrounds. Some will have been raised as children by overprotective parents. Consequently, they may take an excessively cautious attitude towards life. A carer who is overprotective may be reluctant to take any form of risk with clients, no matter how small. This could have serious implications for the autonomy of clients. An overdeveloped sense of safety by carers can result in stifling a client's autonomy by imposing too many petty restrictions.

Alternatively, individuals may rebel against an overprotective childhood by taking reckless risks, both in their personal life and in the way they interact with others. If they become care workers, there is a danger that they will expose clients to unnecessary risks.

In addition to childhood influences, individuals are also affected by other factors, such as the effects of labelling and stereotyping, which can cause them to have beliefs that are detrimental to the welfare of clients.

 Action exercise 2.3

Identify beliefs and influences in your own upbringing, that you feel may have contributed towards your personality. Identify the sources of influence if possible, i.e. parents, friends, teachers or other role models and state how you may have been affected by them

Stereotyping and labelling

The word stereotype originates from the printing industry. Originally it meant a process of preparing a plate of type metal. These days it refers to repetitive and unchanging ideas about people. Stereotypes are broad generalisations. If we describe an Italian, for instance, as someone who is emotional, impulsive, and romantic we are using a stereotype. Another popular myth is that all Germans are hard workers with no sense of humour. These misconceptions happen because personality traits are assigned to a group rather than to an individual.

Differences between the sexes are also susceptible to stereotyping. Words like soft, gentle and delicate are often used to describe feminine attributes. By contrast, masculine characteristics are often depicted as being the opposite of these traits with strength and power being particularly associated with the idea of maleness. In reality, individuals vary tremendously, whether they belong to the same group or not, Not all men are strong or powerful, neither are all women necessarily gentle and weak, and just as there are

Italians who hate pasta, so there are Germans who are lazy but funny.

Although progressive thinking is now challenging some of these broad generalisations, too many people still rely upon them. Stereotyping is a potentially dangerous practice. It convinces us that we understand a person's character and needs, without checking to see if our perceptions are correct. Inevitably this influences the way we behave towards others, as well as how we treat them.

One reason why stereotyping exerts such a powerful influence is because of the labels we attach to people. If a client is labelled 'confused,' there is a danger that staff will perceive that person as being totally helpless and dependent. As a result, carers are likely to make more decisions on behalf of the client, because offering choices to a 'confused' person is seen as a waste of time.

Staff can quickly forget that confused clients can experience episodes of lucid thinking. It is a mistake to regard confusion as being a permanent condition. Even when it is, individuals are still capable of making some decisions for themselves. Unfortunately, once clients are labelled 'confused', they are often denied the opportunity to make decisions.

Objects, as well as people, have labels attached to them. Some serve an extremely useful purpose, like those that identify the contents of a bottle as poison. Labelling people can also be helpful. Describing a group of persons travelling together on a bus as 'passengers' is a convenient way to identify what they have in common. Nevertheless, labels can have the effect of producing negative images.

Even an apparently harmless label like 'passenger' can have a negative meaning. Describing a player in a football match as a 'passenger' suggests that the person is not contributing fully to their team's efforts. The label is negative because it is critical of somebody's apparent lack of effort. It is potentially unfair to the player, because it fails to question if there are reasons to explain his or her poor performance, even though genuine reasons, ranging from injury to lack of match practice, could be responsible.

Labels have the power to influence people. A person who does not pull his or her weight in a group effort is likely to be unpopular. They can become targets for abuse, or experience rejection. Clients in particular often risk being negatively labelled. A common example is when they are labelled 'attention seeking'. This invites carers to dismiss the behaviour of some clients as not worthy of investigation. Consequently they ignore it, just as adults ignore a child's tantrum or an exhibition of showing off.

Treating clients as if they are children, or worse still ignoring them, is not an acceptable standard of care. Discovering the reasons why people behave as they do is more important than simply labelling the behaviour they display.

Labels can be positive as well as negative. The label 'carer' or 'nurse' can conjure up images of an unselfish, devoted person whose main concern is meeting the needs of vulnerable people. While this may reflect a true picture of some carers, it is not an accurate representation of them all. Positive labels can sometimes be just as misleading as negative ones.

Changing perceptions of labels

The messages that labels give out can change over time. Before the Second World War people with learning difficulties were given appalling labels, such as, 'feeble-minded', 'idiot' or 'imbecile'. After changes in mental health law, these offensive names were gradually replaced by the label 'mental subnormality'. This was hardly an improvement, especially for those living in large institutions. The word and image of 'subnormality' became associated with 'sub-humanity'. Even supposedly professional staff were sometimes guilty of referring to clients with severe learning difficulties as 'low grades'.

Attitudes towards clients, who were portrayed as an inferior type of life form, were predictable. In some cases this led to a series of scandals involving the ill treatment of patients in mental institutions. The publicity arising from the scandals eventually led to policy changes. Plans were made to close large institutions and discharge the inmates into the community. At the same time, the expression 'mental subnormality' gradually gave way to a new label: 'mental handicap'.

At first the new label was seen as an improvement upon the old. However, the term 'mental handicap' gradually fell out of favour. The label focused too much on an individual's handicap, rather than upon the individual as a person. Thus, from being a relatively positive label, it became a negative one, which is why today people prefer to use the terms, 'learning disability' or 'learning difficulties'.

Negative labels, such as 'geriatric', 'epileptic' and 'retarded', are also gradually disappearing from everyday use. This is generally a good thing, providing that the labels that replace them are positive and remain so. It is particularly important for carers to discover which labels, if any, are acceptable to their clients. Not everyone in their seventies or eighties wants a label describing them as 'elderly', and some people, although they have a hearing loss, may not wish to be referred to as 'deaf'. People want to be recognised as individuals with a number of dimensions to their personality. They do not want to have undue attention drawn to a particular aspect of their identity which is associated with disadvantage or disability.

Currently, there is a move to replace some existing labels with ones that are more politically correct. This is done in an attempt to overcome racial, sexual and other forms of discrimination. Sometimes the changes meet with popular approval, but not always. Although the public might agree that 'chairperson' is preferable to 'chairman', it does not mean that they welcome every suggestion for change. Some proposals for new alternatives, however, are too radical for people to accept easily into their everyday language.

Even when it is possible to successfully alter labels, the old stereotypes do not disappear overnight. Unless public knowledge increases at the same time, the replacement labels will gradually acquire the same stigmas as the original ones.

Care staff have a crucial role in educating the public, not by formal teaching, but by correcting false impressions concerning clients. When asked about their job, care staff can do much to promote a more positive image of their clients by pointing out many of the myths and stereotypes that surround the client group.

Care staff quickly learn that not all clients become more confused as they get older, or that people suffering from a mental illness necessarily pose any more of a threat to public safety than so-called normal individuals. If they can get these messages across to the general public, it will help reduce many of the stigmas that people attach to vulnerable individuals.

Action exercise 2.4

Make a list of labels attached to people which you think the public regard as negative. Discuss what images are associated with the labels and why they are seen as being negative.

Due to the risk of personal prejudice arising from the effects of stereotyping or negative labelling, important ethical decisions are best made in conjunction with other people. Everyone, including relatives, other staff members, voluntary helpers and, not least the clients themselves, should have an opportunity to put their views forward.

Senior managers, who may be to some extent removed from regular close involvement with clients, should seek the views of everyone concerned in the care process. This is to ensure that there is a full debate over issues affecting the fair treatment of individual clients.

To contribute to the discussions, care staff require some understanding of ethical theory, principles and practices. Without such an understanding, there is always the risk that decisions about care will be made in the interests of staff rather than clients.

Case study

Rodney is a 60-year-old man with learning difficulties. He has recently been discharged from a long stay hospital in which he spent over 40 years. He now lives in a staff-supported four-bedded house in the community. He continues to wear a hat bought many years ago on an outing to the seaside. It bears the inscription 'kiss me quick'. Because staff think that people are laughing at him they try to persuade him not to wear the hat in public. He is extremely reluctant to surrender his cherished possession, especially as he wore it for years in the secluded grounds of the hospital. He bursts into tears at the thought that he might not be able to wear the hat. Discuss this situation and decide what, if anything, you will do to prevent him from being publicly ridiculed.

Summary of key points

- The extent to which people's needs are satisfied is a measure of the quality of their life.

- Care staff should be aware of the dangers which abrupt changes in lifestyle can have on their client's health and needs.
- A justification for overruling a client's wishes is when doing so avoids causing harm to the individual or to other people.
- Acting paternalistically means taking decisions on behalf of clients to promote their welfare.
- When paternalistic decisions are taken on behalf of clients, attempts should be made to promote their future autonomy as much as possible.
- Utilitarianism is an ethical theory which attempts to measure the rightness of an action by the number of people who benefit by it.
- A disadvantage of utilitarianism is that it often ignores minority interests.
- Paternalistic decisions should not be made by carers acting alone.
- The effect of stereotyping and negative labelling can prevent carers from seeing clients as individuals and treating them as such.
- Carers have a role in educating the public to see clients as individuals in their own right.

Chapter 3
Equality and Rights

Rights and responsibilities

In democratic countries there is wide recognition that individuals possess certain basic human and moral rights. Consequently, there is public concern if things such as rights to privacy, safety, information, employment, education and health care are not upheld. A part of a care-worker's role is to ensure that their clients receive fair treatment as well as the rights due to them. Consequently, it is useful for carers to have some understanding of rights and of their corresponding responsibilities.

Rights are normally described as justified entitlements that are held equally by everyone. There are two major categories of rights: moral and legal, although the distinctions between the two are not always clear-cut.

Those which are enforceable by acts of parliament or common law are legal rights. They cover a variety of different things, ranging from the way in which people behave, to the products that they buy. As consumers, any goods we purchase must be of a reasonable quality; if not we can demand a refund. If a retailer refuses to reimburse us, we can ask a civil court to invoke the law.

Similarly, legal rights exist to protect people from harassment or discrimination. If individuals experience unfair treatment they can apply to a court or body, such as the Commission for Racial Equality, for a ruling that will safeguard their rights. By comparison, the lack of a legal framework makes moral rights less easy to secure, sometimes to such a degree that some people even question the usefulness of them, believing instead that the only rights worth having are legal ones.

Moral rights are those that have developed over the years and entered the belief system of a democratic society. The freedom to speak openly is an example of one that is cherished in the UK. Sometimes, an entitlement starts out as a moral right but in time becomes a legal one.

One of the most generally accepted moral rights is a right to life itself. From the time that child labour was used in Victorian factories, humanitarians have argued that workers had a moral right to protection from the dangers of the workplace. Today, that moral right has, in some areas of life, become a legal one. Employees now have health and safety at work legislation to protect them on the shop floor.

Some of the rights relevant to clients have already been mentioned, like the right to openly express wishes, opinions and beliefs. This particular entitlement comes under the general heading of freedom of speech. However, rights are not without restrictions: they also bring with them responsibilities. For example, although both clients and carers have a right to speak freely, they also have a corresponding duty to speak responsibly.

There are limits to what we can say about people in public. For example, it is neither morally nor legally justifiable to make inflammatory racial or religious remarks. Similarly, without any supporting evidence, it is irresponsible and against the law to slander people. Rights are only justified, providing those claiming them accept the responsibilities which accompany them.

 Action exercise 3.1 _____

Discuss some of the moral or human rights that you believe you are entitled to. Also, identify any responsibilities that you think accompany those particular rights.

Characteristics of moral rights

Rights are sometimes also classified as being either positive or negative. The difference between the two depends upon the type of duty that each demands. Every time a person claims a positive right, someone else has to carry out a specific duty. Rights to welfare are examples of positive rights. A doctor, a chief executive of a health authority or a care worker, has a duty to provide welfare services to the person who is claiming a right to health care.

Negative rights, by contrast, only require others not to interfere. These rights are sometimes referred to as liberty rights. When people say 'It's a free country, isn't it?' they are usually referring to negative, or liberty rights. Living in a democratic society means that, within reason, people are free to speak their minds or move around the country at will. Providing people keep within the law, the only duty that negative rights demand is that others should not try to prevent individuals from speaking their minds, or interfere with their movements.

Rights are not absolute. This means that there are occasions when it is possible to legitimately overrule them. The right to life is one of the most important rights that people cherish, but despite this there are times when it is permissible to take the life of another individual. The most common justification for taking a life is when a person has to act in self-defence.

It might not be possible to obtain some rights because of a lack of resources. For example, clients have privacy rights. If they live in a care home where bedrooms are shared they could claim that, on privacy grounds, they have a right to a room of their own. If no single rooms are available, however, it is impossible to meet this particular demand.

Nevertheless staff should observe their client's privacy as much as possible, especially when clients are dressing, bathing or engaging in other intimate activities. Although clients cannot always obtain all their privacy rights, it is important that they get as many as possible. If necessary, adaptations to the environment should be made to achieve this end.

Although rights are considered to be equal, the way in which they are exercised may not be. Personal hygiene, for instance, is an essential requirement of daily life, and to deprive clients of opportunities to wash makes them more susceptible to possible infections. All clients have a right to have access to washing facilities to protect them from possible diseases. Dependent clients however require more. They need staff assistance to exercise their rights to protect their health. The aid required may range from a little help with shampooing of their hair, to being entirely bathed by staff. Consequently, although in principle rights are equal, there can be inequalities in the manner in which they are exercised.

In addition, although rights belong to everybody equally, at least in theory, people are not equal. There can be tremendous differences between individuals, for example, some being stronger than others, or more wealthy or more intelligent. Inequalities exist between people's environments and their genetic make-up.

Even in a residential care home where all the clients may be elderly or have learning difficulties, the differences can still be seen. Some clients will be much more withdrawn than others, or more excitable; some will have a limited ability to speak or communicate; others will have additional mental or sensory handicaps which make it harder for them to claim their rights. Since these differences often have the effect of making it particularly difficult for disadvantaged people to claim their entitlements, some people argue that a system of equal rights is not necessarily a fair one. Consequently, a case is sometimes advanced that rights should take account of these differences and discriminate in favour of people who are particularly disadvantaged.

Conflicts between rights

In the United States programmes of positive discrimination exist to make up for the lack of opportunities that many disadvantaged groups experience. In some regions, black people are given preferential treatment when applying for jobs and for places at university. In these cases, the law demands that employers and colleges take a certain number of applicants, regardless of whether their qualifications are inferior to those of other white candidates.

These programmes positively discriminate in favour of disadvantaged groups, in the hope of raising their standards of living and education. It is an inescapable fact that many have suffered the most abject poverty, living in slum dwellings with their children attending the most deprived schools. The expectation is that, in time, these groups will become as affluent as the existing white population.

However, discriminatory rights have caused both conflicts and bitterness. Disappointed white applicants argue that positive discrimination is unfair to them. Some argue that there is little point in obtaining better qualifications, if they are refused places at university or rejected at job interviews in favour of those who are relatively poorly qualified. They accuse the policy of being unjust as it makes them personally responsible for the past racial injustices of earlier white generations.

Whatever the merits or disadvantages of positive discrimination, it does focus attention on the need for fairness in society. In the UK a form of positive discrimination also exists. For many years businesses employing 20 or more workers have had to reserve, by law, a number of jobs for people with disabilities. Certain occupations, such as lift or car park attendants, are sometimes kept open specifically for this purpose. Unfortunately, many employers have been guilty of disregarding the regulations. The Disability Discrimination Act 1995 aims to bring about future improvements for people with disabilities.

 Action exercise 3.2 _____

If a programme of positive discrimination for vulnerable people was instituted in the UK, discuss which areas the programme should address and whether the advantages of the programme would outweigh any disadvantages.

Conflicts about a client's rights can arise in care homes as they can anywhere else, but merely claiming a moral right is unlikely to bring about an end to conflict. If two clients want to view different television programmes at the same time, and only one set is available, there is little point in them appealing to rights. Both clients have an equal claim to be free to enjoy their leisure time as they wish. Equality means that one person's rights are no more important than anyone else's.

In recent years many long-stay institutions have closed, which were home to people with learning difficulties. Many former inmates are now exercising their entitlement to live in the community. However, some are already discovering the limitations of rights. Moving out of an institution is only a beginning. Unless individuals can integrate into their local community, they risk facing the same amount of isolation in their new life, as they did in their old.

Although there are rights for individuals to have the opportunity to integrate into society, there is no right to integrate: not if rights are equal. People value the freedom to choose their own friends and companions, also, the freedom to ignore those with whom they have little in common. There is a conflict between the aim to integrate people into society and the rights of people in society to determine with whom they want to integrate.

Most of us interact with people of similar interests. If we like sport then probably most of our friends like sport too. If we are bored by politics, it is unlikely that we will opt to spend much time with politicians. Consequently, moral rights cannot force a policy of integration upon society. Valuable as rights are, they also have their limitations. In the case of clients with learning difficulties, although integration is not a right, carers should do everything they can to provide clients with ample opportunities to join in the activities of the local community.

Duties

Conflicts between competing rights are not uncommon. Care workers have a duty to ensure that all residents are treated fairly and to search for solutions when conflicts arise. There are important differences between rights and duties. The differences are significant because whereas rights do not have to be exercised, duties must be carried out.

Servicemen who fail to carry out their duties during war face court martial and even the death penalty. In peacetime, employees risk a disciplinary interview or dismissal for lapses of duty at work. By contrast, individuals do not have to exercise their rights.

Although people have a right to a freedom of speech, they can choose to stay silent if they wish. Similarly, having a right to health care does not mean that a person has to see a doctor when ill. People can choose whether to exercise a right or refrain from doing so. Duties are different: they have to be undertaken, unless exceptional circumstances exist which justify a reason not to. This has important implications for staff. Many clients are vulnerable people who are unable to easily obtain their rights and thus staff have to assist them, whether a client chooses to exercise a specific right or not. However, clients have a right to complain about ill treatment. In some situations they may refrain from exercising this right, fearing that a complaint may only make matters worse for them. If a member of staff sees another carer abusing a client they *must* report the matter to a senior colleague. This is because it is a duty and unlike a right, there is no alternative.

Just as conflicts between rights can sometimes arise, so too can conflicts between duties. Communal living can lower tolerance levels between clients and petty irritations can erupt into full-blown quarrels. Care staff have a duty to help clients resolve their differences, especially if other residents are being adversely affected by them.

Confused clients can act irrationally at times. There may be occasions when they make disparaging personal remarks about other clients, not because of deliberate malice, but because of their mental state. Staff have a duty to protect the clients who are the victims of the verbal abuse, as well as the person responsible for making the comments. The way in which staff achieve this will vary according to the circumstances. The key ethical principle involved in the above example is avoiding harm. Although clients, like staff, have a right to freedom of speech, it does not extend to making malicious public remarks about other people. The victim of a verbal assault requires protection. Staff also have to find acceptable ways to prevent the client responsible from continuing the verbal abuse. They have to see that the abuser is treated fairly and with respect, especially as he or she may not be aware of the hurt that they are causing.

Challenging behaviours

Sometimes, it is possible to discover why individuals behave in a way that is distressing to others. In some cases boredom, or a general lack of stimulation, can act as a trigger for someone to become aggressive either physically or verbally. The provision of a more stimulating environment can significantly reduce the likelihood of such outbursts for those clients who have a low boredom threshold.

Another possible cause of irritable behaviour can be due to physical factors, such as decreased blood sugar levels. Clients most likely to be affected are those with poor early morning appetites who eat little or nothing at breakfast. Something as simple as a mid-morning snack can help maintain these clients in a more tranquil state of mind.

Many other factors are potential sources of annoyance to residents. If carers can identify them and take measures to prevent them from triggering antisocial behaviours, this will reduce the likelihood of disruption and harm occurring to the client group.

However, it is not always possible to find logical reasons to explain why individuals behave in a certain way, particularly if the person concerned is confused. Staff who are unable to find reasons to account for a client's behaviour are still left with the task of ensuring that no major harm occurs to the individual or to the remaining residents.

If an abusive individual continues to make unreasonable verbal assaults on fellow residents, despite pleas to stop, it may be necessary to employ different strategies. Sometimes it is possible to divert someone from a particular behaviour pattern by interesting him or her in an alternative one. Merely changing the subject by asking a question can sometimes work, particularly if the question relates to a personal interest.

Diversions can sometimes be achieved by offers of alternative occupation or recreation. However, offers such as 'Would you like to go for a walk, Mr X?' or 'Can you help me finish this jigsaw puzzle, Mrs Y?' are only likely to be effective if they are activities which the client genuinely enjoys.

These strategies will not always be successful. However, from an ethical viewpoint they attempt to minimise the harm to the victims of the verbal abuse, while at the same time respecting the needs of the individual who is unintentionally responsible for the situation.

Sometimes, when diversionary tactics fail to work, it is necessary to protect the client group by temporarily removing the disturbed client from the immediate environment. This is sometimes known as time-out. They may have to be taken to their bedroom or some quiet corner. If an individual does have to be excluded from interacting with fellow residents, it must be for therapeutic reasons and not punitive ones.

A therapeutic intervention is one that allows a disruptive client the opportunity to be in quiet surroundings away from the focus of his or her irritation – in this case, those clients who are the subjects of the abuse.

Clients in temporary exclusion should never be left alone. At all times a carer should accompany them, preferably one with whom they have had an opportunity to build up a relationship. The carer's role is to provide support and to reassure the client that exclusion is not a punishment.

Even when clients are confused they are still entitled to explanations. Staff can point out that it is quite normal, even in close families, for people to get on each other's nerves. And that until tempers cool, it is often best if those arguing can distance themselves from each other for a while and take a quiet break. Establishments should always have policies governing time-out procedures and they should be reviewed regularly.

The management of challenging behaviour

Fear, whether real or imagined, can spark off anger. Clients who exhibit disruptive behaviour may be experiencing irrational fears. Care staff should try to demonstrate concern, warmth and reassurance with any clients they temporarily exclude because of disturbed behaviour. Time-out procedures should be as brief as possible. As soon as an individual is suitably calm, staff should ask whether he or she feels ready to rejoin the rest of the group.

During a client's exclusion, other care staff have the responsibility for attending to the emotions and needs of the remaining clients. Staff should point out to those who have been verbally abused, that the offender is not responsible for his or her actions and persuade them not to hold grudges. By monitoring the situation, when an individual returns from a period of exclusion, staff can ensure that a repetition of disruptive behaviour does not immediately occur. Staff may have to also apply other strategies such as finding more effective ways to occupy a client, or adapting the environment to reduce anxiety levels or potential sources of irritation.

Methods of dealing with ethical dilemmas will vary according to individual circumstances. However, an essential first step in finding a morally justifiable solution is to identify which ethical principles are involved and to use them as a basis for decision making.

Action exercise 3.3 _____

Make a list of things or situations that cause personal anxiety or fear. Briefly describe how you react to fearful situations both mentally and physically. State what, if anything, helps you cope with anxiety. By discussion, compare which fears and coping strategies are common within the group, and which are not.

Sometimes, it is not clients who are the targets of verbal abuse but members of staff. Although their feelings may be hurt, they have the responsibility of retaining their composure. When staff are first recruited, they should be made aware that part of their duties will involve working with some individuals who at times exhibit difficult behaviour. This places staff into a different category from clients. To them a residential home is a workplace. They voluntarily accept any potential disruptions that may occur within it as part of the job for which they are paid.

In contrast, a residential establishment is home for the clients who live there. Either directly or indirectly, they pay to live in it and do not expect to have to tolerate difficult behaviour from other people. When individual clients exhibit challenging behaviours, staff have to serve the needs of both the individual under stress, as well as those of the remaining clients. This does not mean that staff have to tolerate any behaviour which is directed towards them, no matter how extreme. They too have rights to protection and needs that must be met. We shall look at some of these in a later chapter. For now it is sufficient to say that staff require training on how to react to displays of threatening behaviour, and support to cope with stresses that their job might cause.

Distributive justice and resource allocation

Rights are important, but, treating people fairly can sometimes be more important than treating them equally. The way in which resources are distributed is crucial in the provision of health and social care. Resources are finite, not limitless. Consequently, allocations need to be fair so that some people do not have a lion's share, while others have none. Justice is the ethical principle concerned with fairness, and distributive justice simply means allocating goods and services fairly.

Most people resent unfair practices, which is why individuals who attempt to push their way into a queue are unpopular. Rules exist to ensure that people wait their turn. Usually, there is general agreement that those who have been queuing the longest time deserve serving first. However, there may be genuine reasons why this may not always be the case.

In the field of health care, patients awaiting operations normally have to join a waiting list before their turn for treatment comes. Despite this, some patients who are victims of a heart attack or a road traffic accident are admitted to hospital for emergency care ahead of those already in a queue for surgery. People accept queue jumping of this kind because they agree that the needs of someone in a medical emergency require urgent attention. Individuals also know that if their own life is similarly at risk, they too will receive priority emergency treatment. Thus, although it is not always possible to distribute resources equally, efforts should be made to allocate them fairly.

There are many different types of resources, and because they are scarce staff have to be careful how they distribute them. Resources such as the buildings that house the clients, or the furnishings and equipment within, are not likely to involve staff in making decisions on the allocation of assets. Although, as we saw earlier in the dispute about the television, conflicts can arise when these type of resources are limited.

The most important resources are the quantity and quality of staff who serve the needs of the clients. The amount of time that can be spent with each client is dependent upon the number of staff available, as well as upon their levels of skill and experience. While staff are serving the needs of some clients, inevitably there will be others who are left unattended. The problem for carers is to allocate their time as fairly as possible.

Reaching an agreement on what is fair is not always easy. Many years ago, a now famous piece of research was undertaken by a nurse called Felicity Stockwell. The study demonstrated that some hospital patients were unpopular with staff and consequently received considerably less nursing attention than other more 'likeable' patients. Patients who made complaints or who were more critical of their care were particularly unpopular with staff.

The results of this research study were not really very surprising. Most of us prefer to be in the company of people whom we like. However, the job of care staff is to serve the needs of vulnerable individuals, regardless of whether they are likeable or not.

Sometimes, as we have seen, there are reasons why some clients deserve more attention than others. However, it is never justifiable for carers to allocate the amount of time spent with clients according to their own personal preferences. This is why, when time is short, staff must consider the fairest way to distribute it.

One way to distribute resources is according to need. The difficulty with this approach is that sometimes it is hard to measure one person's needs against those of another. It is comparatively easy to see that a client who is dependent upon staff for washing or feeding will have the greater need than those who are able to do these things for themselves. But as discussed earlier, individuals have a wide variety of needs and they tend to view their own as being particularly important.

Less dependent clients will have other needs that require fulfilling. They will want to interact with staff, whether just for light-hearted banter or because they have anxieties they want to discuss. They too will want staff attention. The problem for carers, when there is not enough time in the day, or insufficient staff on duty, is how to make the fairest use of the time available.

The process of institutionalisation

Carers usually overcome this problem by prioritising needs, with those necessary for survival being given priority. Staff usually first attend to dependent clients who require feeding, bathing and washing. However, the burden of fulfilling the physical needs of many severely dependent clients can be overwhelming. By the time all the clients have been fed, washed and dressed, the staff themselves are sometimes exhausted. It is tempting then to sit clients passively in front of a television set while carers take a well-earned break themselves.

Naturally, staff require breaks during the working day, but

sometimes there is a tendency for everyone to have their breaks at the same time. Although socially rewarding for them, it is at the cost of leaving clients sitting neglected in isolation. Managers have to help staff find a balance between the workload necessary to satisfy the physical requirements of some clients and that required to meet the mental and emotional needs of others.

It is quite normal for staff in the workplace to adopt a routine approach to the outstanding tasks of the day. People in their own homes tend to do certain things at set times. In many homes the times of family meals do not usually vary by a great deal, neither do the times for getting up and going to bed, at least during the working week.

Daily routines can help people organise their time more effectively. However, carried to an extreme, routines can become monotonous, unstimulating and lead to institutionalisation.

This is a process in which people living under a rigid routine have their needs attended to *en masse*, rather than individually. Everyone is fed or dressed at the same time, or washed and bathed together. Institutionalisation subjects people to a system of block treatment which exerts tremendous control over their lives. Consequently, they become resigned to a passive acceptance of the daily routines that are imposed upon them. This often results in apathy and a loss of personal identity.

Institutionalisation also affects staff, although in a different way. They become used to seeing people not as individuals but as representing units of work. Like an assembly line in a factory, so many bodies have to be processed each day – that is fed, cleansed, dressed and changed. Quality of care gives way to productivity. The worker who can bathe the most clients in the quickest time becomes viewed as being the most efficient. Communication tends to be reduced to staff ordering clients to comply with the routine tasks that have to be undertaken. Many of the worst aspects of care, which were highlighted in past scandals involving long-stay hospitals, came about because of the institutionalisation process which was responsible for dehumanising both staff and clients alike.

Action exercise 3.4 _____

Draw up a list of activities in your life which are subject to more or less the same routine and those which are not. Discuss how you feel about routines that are imposed upon you by circumstances beyond your control and those which you voluntarily choose to adopt.

Staff, therefore, have the difficult task of attending to clients in the fairest way possible, bearing in mind that time is usually in short supply. Carers often have to prioritise client's needs, with basic ones being attended to first, but at the same time not forgetting that the requirements of less dependent clients also have to be satisfied.

In attending to needs, carers have to make certain that they do not lapse into the rigid routines discussed in the institutionalisation process. Consequently, it is not only important to distribute resources fairly; the manner in which they are distributed can be equally crucial.

Case study _____

Jody is a young man of 18 who has learning difficulties. Because of illness his mother can no longer care for him at home. Recently he has moved into a staff-supported house with three other young male clients. Jody neglects his personal hygiene and his fellow tenants complain to him and to staff that he is 'dirty and smelly'. Discuss how staff might tackle this problem.

Summary of key points

- Moral rights are justified entitlements equally due to everyone.
- Legal rights, unlike moral rights, are enforceable by acts of parliament or common law.
- Rights carry with them responsibilities which have to be discharged.
- A positive right requires another person or persons to carry out specific duties.
- A negative right requires only that others do not interfere.
- Clients may need additional assistance from carers to claim their rights.

- Duties are obligations which must be carried out, in contrast to rights which may or may not be exercised.
- Conflicts can arise between clients claiming equal rights which need to be resolved by staff.
- There are occasions when rights can be justifiably overridden.

Chapter 4
Communication and Advocacy

Importance of effective communication

The way in which people communicate gives an indication of the amount of respect they have for each other. People who yell and shout are obviously not demonstrating much in the way of mutual regard. The quality of any relationship between two individuals depends, to a large extent, upon an effective system of communication, which is why care staff should strive to become proficient in their interactions with clients.

Staff have to be able to communicate effectively with clients to discover their wishes and requirements, but communication is important for reasons other than just to exchange factual information. People feel a need to communicate their feelings to others close to them, especially when they are anxious or fearful. At such times they seek reassurance and comfort, to put their minds at rest.

Clients have these same needs for trust and security, which have to be met. Consequently, carers who are competent at communicating are in a better position to help them. Sometimes barriers to effective communication have to be overcome before meaningful interaction can take place between clients and carers.

A number of obstacles can make communication difficult. Sight and hearing can deteriorate as clients grow older, adversely affecting their reading and listening skills. In some cases, the provision of glasses or hearing aids may be all that is necessary.

The situation is more serious, however, if an individual becomes totally blind or deaf. As a person grows older, learning new skills becomes more difficult. For a young person, learning Braille might be comparatively simple, but it becomes progressively harder as the years advance and concentration spans decline.

It can be particularly difficult communicating with clients who suffer from confusion, or a mental illness which causes them to hear voices or experience similar hallucinations. Many of these clients, however, will have some episodes when things are clear enough for them to understand simple messages.

Other factors besides physical ones can make communicating difficult. People under a lot of stress, or in a highly charged emotional state, are sometimes unable to grasp the meaning of traumatic news. An unwelcome message like the report of the death of a loved one, or the birth of a baby with a serious handicap, can be met with total disbelief. This refusal to believe bad news is known as a state of denial and can prove a serious block to effective communication.

Action exercise 4.1

Identify factors that could be barriers to communication besides the ones mentioned in the text. Discuss how some of these might be overcome or their effects minimised.

Although speech is the commonest form of communication, it is only one of several methods. Facial expression, as well as the way that people hold and position their body, give clues to their moods and feelings. Usually it is possible to tell when someone is angry, frightened or sad, just by looking at them. Since some clients will not have any meaningful speech, staff have to become proficient in recognising and interpreting body language messages.

People from different cultures vary in the body language that they use. For some, standing too close can cause acute discomfort, especially if they are born into a society which values a large amount of personal space compared with other cultures. Similarly, maintaining eye contact is more valued in some societies than others. While some communities consider it rude to maintain eye contact, except for the briefest of moments, others believe that avoiding eye contact is a sign of mistrust. Therefore, staff should be aware of these differences, particularly if they are caring for clients from a different ethnic background to their own.

If a carer's initial form of communication is not effective, he or she will have to try alternative approaches. These can range from approved sign languages, such as British Sign Language or Makaton, to informal ones, designed specifically to meet the requirements of particular clients.

Such is the speed of progress of microchip technology that a huge range of new communication devices and software are constantly appearing. Consequently, care workers are likely to need increased training in communications technology in the future, in order to make the most efficient use of the resources available.

Problems with communicating

Despite the appearance of sophisticated communication hardware, one of the most powerful forms of communication is human touch. Holding a person's hand or putting a protective arm around their shoulder can provide feelings of reassurance to someone who is anxious or frightened; especially if they are unable to understand spoken words of comfort.

However, some individuals are more reserved than others and do not welcome displays of public emotion. Other than an introductory handshake, some clients would probably prefer to avoid close physical contact with strangers. It is helpful if staff know their client's attitudes towards touching – a hug that is friendly to some may be quite the opposite to others.

Unwanted and unexpected physical contact can lead to accusations of abuse, assault or even sexual harassment. People usually have to form a reasonably close relationship with each other before they are ready to communicate by touch, although there are always exceptions. Some individuals are much less inhibited than others and will not shrink from making physical contact even with comparative strangers.

The difficulty for clients and care staff is that intimate contact sometimes has to take place before either have had a chance to form a close relationship. Someone who requires help in bathing or dressing has little choice but to submit to some form of physical contact from a carer. Staff can reduce the effects of the unwelcome experience for the client by ensuring privacy and explaining what is about to happen.

By contrast, there are some individuals who positively welcome close contact with their carers. A number of adult clients with learning difficulties, for instance, will happily grasp a carer's arm when out in public, even when they are capable of walking unaided. This matters little if the client is an elderly person, but the public tend to look twice if the client is a young adult, or a man of middle years. They see it as a sign that these people are different from the norm, because in this country, men are not normally seen linking arms or holding hands in public.

Unfortunately, a person who stands out as being different from others has a much harder task of being accepted into society. The way an individual behaves communicates certain messages to other people. As part of the caring role is to promote opportunities for clients with learning disabilities to integrate into society, it can be in the interests of some clients to dissuade them from inappropriate public displays of affection or physical contact.

However, if physical contact is necessary to protect a client from potential harm it must be given, regardless of whether or not it singles them out for public attention. A person who cannot cross the road, for instance, clearly requires the support of a carer.

It is not only people with learning disabilities who have problems with integration. People can change, and so can their circumstances. The onset of a mental illness or confusion in old age can affect the way that others interact with an individual. Someone previously well regarded by their peers can, through no fault of their own, find themselves viewed with less value. They are no longer held in respect, because their condition creates stigmas and causes them to lose social status in the eyes of an unthinking public.

Principle of normalisation

In the field of learning disabilities a philosophy prevails which attempts to present individuals in a more valued light. Known originally as normalisation, it aims to improve the integration of this group of people into society. It is critical of the way the public communicates with these disadvantaged people. The philosophy also criticises those who 'talk down' to disadvantaged people, or treat them in other childish ways. Elderly persons often experience similar treatment.

Addressing adults as if they are children singles them out as being different from 'normal' people. Instead of respecting them as valued citizens, society views them with negative emotions, such as fear or pity. The principles of normalisation have evolved over the years to become known, rather dauntingly, as social role valorisation (SRV). However, the major aim of the philosophy is to correct society's attitudes by improving the image that devalued people present to the world.

Critics of normalisation argue that it is a philosophy which concentrates upon moulding an individual to fit into society's values, without questioning whether the values are worth adopting. Whether carers agree with the philosophy or not, they should make sure that they try to address clients appropriately when communicating with them.

There will be times when it is impossible to communicate with a client exactly as one would with another adult of the same age. Consequently staff may have to use a different strategy to get their meaning across. Even childish methods can be justified if they are the only way to ensure that communication with a particular client is effective, although such methods should be regarded as the exception rather than the rule.

 Action exercise 4.2 _____

Identify ways in which people communicate messages of disrespect to other individuals and groups or show by their attitude that they hold them in low esteem.

Advocacy – the role of the care worker

Carers have a number of key duties to undertake in the area of communication. To establish a relationship with their client they first have to set up a communication system with them. Many times this will be comparatively simple, requiring only the abilities to listen actively and to speak clearly at a level that the client understands.

At other times, establishing a communication system will be more difficult and it may be necessary to employ a system of signs or symbols. We have seen an important part of a carer's duties is to encourage clients to express their wishes and beliefs to promote their autonomy. Unfortunately, a few individuals will be unable to express their preferences and consequently will require the help of someone who can speak for them.

Without the services of an advocate, clients who are unable to make their own voices heard are in danger of losing their rights. Advocacy is consequently an integral part of any system of communication between clients and carers. Many clients are able to be their own self-advocate and are articulate enough to claim their rights and express their opinions. However, those unable to do this need the services of another person to act as a citizen advocate to speak on their behalf and preserve their interests.

If staff take on this role, they first have to build up a relationship of trust with the clients. It is the key to effective communication. Other skills are also required, such as the ability to express oneself clearly, and to receive, interpret and comprehend messages. However, no matter how adept people are in these skills, unless they can convince others that they are trustworthy, the messages they communicate are likely to be less than effective.

People tend to be wary about confiding in individuals that they do not trust. If a client feels that a particular carer is untrustworthy, then almost certainly some communication problems will exist between them. For example, a carer may clearly explain to a resident that it is time to take their medicine and the client may experience no problem in understanding the message. However, if trust is missing, or the client is suspicious of the carer's motives, they may refuse to take their prescribed drugs.

Whether clients require advocacy on a temporary or permanent basis will depend upon their circumstances, which in turn affects the role of the staff. Someone who suffers a stroke and loses their power of speech will almost certainly want the help of an advocate. However, sometimes clients can make rapid recoveries from a stroke. Consequently, if they are able to resume communicating, then staff can gradually withdraw from the advocate role.

There are reasons other than illness or handicap, which can inhibit individuals from being self-advocates. Former inmates of long stay hospitals may have been deprived of chances of speaking up for themselves. Institutionalisation tends to stifle autonomy and restrict opportunities for exercising personal choice. Therefore, a key part of the role of present-day care workers is to teach institu-tionalised clients how to make their voices heard.

The best way to achieve this is to offer clients the opportunity to make choices whenever possible. Regularly exposing them to the decision-making process will improve their competence in forming judgements. If some decisions are potentially too risky, staff will still have to continue to exercise judgement on their behalf, until they acquire a measure of proficiency.

For example, it is in the interests of clients to make sure that they are aware of safe practices before encouraging them to use a cooker to prepare a meal. However, the overall aim should be to extend the client's range of skills and experiences to provide the autonomy required to become their own self-advocates.

Constraints to effective listening

Helping clients to speak for themselves requires staff to become active listeners. There is little point in providing clients with the confidence to communicate, if staff then fail to listen properly to what they have to say. Much of the time people only half listen to what is said. They are often too busy thinking instead of what they are going to say next. Consequently, many misunderstandings arise which adversely affect the quality of the communication process. To avoid these pitfalls, staff should try to cultivate the habit of active listening.

Active listening is an exacting occupation. It demands full con-centration upon the words being uttered and upon their meaning. Often supplementary questions need to be asked to clarify what someone is saying. A client who exclaims 'I think I will go to bed now,' may do so because they feel tired, whereas another client might make the same comment because there is nothing else to do. It is important to know the thoughts behind the words. If lack of stimulation is causing an individual to retire early, then the client is really communicating that he or she is bored, in which case, staff should make an effort to interest them in some useful occupation.

Active listening calls for the mental questioning of the meaning of someone else's words. If uncertainty about their meaning still persists, then questions in the mind can be spoken aloud. Active listening is time consuming because it requires concentration, and sometimes it is necessary to ask further questions. Therefore there has to be sufficient time available to practise it. Staff who are working busily on a variety of different tasks are unlikely to be able to listen effectively. On these occasions conversation is more likely to be general and superficial.

There are other restraints to effective listening to consider. Clients may be tired or simply not in a talkative frame of mind. Staff must respect not only the wishes of the clients but their moods too. Communication is a two-way process and if an individual is reluctant to participate then it is largely ineffective.

Sometimes the immediate environment may not be suitable for what a client wishes to say. A day room where a number of other residents are within earshot clearly lacks privacy. The need to preserve confidentiality will be discussed in more detail later. However, staff should be aware that a lack of privacy, in some circumstances, can be a potential restraint to effective communication.

There are a number of possible reasons why some clients may be unable to speak for themselves. An individual with a very severe learning disability may never have had the intellectual capacity to understand the issues that affect his or her life. A client experiencing this degree of handicap may need an advocate permanently.

 Action exercise 4.3 _____

Discuss the following:

As well as being an active listener, what other qualities or characteristics does an advocate need to possess in order to be effective when speaking on behalf of another individual?

Who should be an advocate?

The question of who is the best person to act as an advocate for clients is a complex one. Opinions are divided on the matter. In hospitals and nursing homes, many qualified nurses, for instance, argue that they should take on the role. They cite the fact that they are subject to a professional code of conduct which demands that they act in the best interests of the patient. They are also on duty and available to provide their services for twenty four hours a day, all year – unlike friends or relatives.

Medical staff make similar claims, since they are also answerable to an ethical code. They too provide services throughout the year and have legal responsibilities of care towards patients. Social workers and other professional staff have also claimed the privilege of acting as an advocate for clients.

However, some people are against the idea of any paid employees acting as advocates. They argue that there can be a clash of interests between the needs of the staff and those of the clients. It might be beneficial, for instance, to have extra staff on duty at weekends or evenings to extend the range of leisure activities available to residents. However, a change of shift pattern affects the personal lives of staff and also those of their partners or families. Consequently, if it is not in the interests of staff to work different hours, it is unlikely that they will be able to argue impartially on behalf of clients.

According to some, the people in the best position to speak on behalf of clients are relatives or close friends. Relatives certainly will know the client much better than a member of staff and have a good idea of the client's likes and dislikes. They will also have the client's best interests at heart, although this is not necessarily always the case.

However, relatives, unlike staff, are not always immediately available when needed. Furthermore, they may not feel competent to act as an advocate or show an interest in doing so.

Perhaps the ideal person to act as an advocate is a volunteer. Compared with either a member of staff or a relative, voluntary workers are independent. They have no axe to grind and there is considerably less chance of them being motivated by self interest. Unfortunately, there is a major difficulty in using volunteers as advocates. It is extremely hard to attract sufficient people who have the ability and the desire to take on the job. If staff know of any suitable people interested in becoming a citizen advocate, they can help their own clients by encouraging likely candidates to come forward.

Staff sometimes have no other option but to act as an advocate for a client, simply because nobody else is available, or wants to take on the role. Most clients receive, as a matter of routine, a high standard of care and their just entitlements. Nevertheless, even in the best run establishments, it is sometimes possible to overlook the interests of a client. Consequently, there will be occasions when someone needs to speak up on behalf of clients and the only person available to do that is a member of staff. A good example of a client needing the services of an advocate is when he or she is penalised for disruptive behaviour. A member of staff is well placed to be an advocate, particularly if no-one else is ready to do so.

Clients are not necessarily deliberately left out of activities by staff. Sometimes, however, carers just assume that a particular person would not enjoy a certain activity, especially if he or she is unable to communicate very well. Consequently, a client may not get a chance to see if they would enjoy a particular experience, which is why it is important that there is someone available to speak up for them.

Truth telling

In all their communications staff should strive to be as honest as possible. Unfortunately, this is not always the case. Sometimes, they practise deceptions, because they feel it is in the client's best interests to do so. On closer examination however, lying is often in their own interests rather than the client's.

A client may become upset because a relative, without notifying anyone, fails to appear on a regular visiting day. It might be comparatively easy to pacify the client with a 'white lie' by telling them that their relative will probably call the following week. As well as calming the client, this may also have the effect of providing staff with respite from the attentions of the distressed individual. But if the staff have no idea whether the visitor will call the following week, then they are acting unethically. If the visitor fails to appear, then the deception has achieved little except to undermine trust. It is better for staff to attempt to discover the real reason for a visitor's absence and communicate it to the client, than invent an elaborate fairy tale. If the reasons are not discoverable, then other methods of placating hurt feelings should be tried instead of lying.

Many of the incidents where staff are tempted to lie to clients may appear to be trivial, although not to the client they affect. Often situations arise where there are no easy answers and whatever staff do, a client will experience some hurt.

Occasionally relatives may not want to remain in contact with a client at all, and ask staff not to continue to send them any more letters or cards from the individual. There can be a number of reasons for this. It may be because the family is emigrating to another country and feel a clean break is the best course of action for all concerned, or it may be that a relative has remarried, and their new partner does not want either of them to maintain the existing family link. Whatever the reason, it poses problems for staff. There are no easy answers to ethical dilemmas and often all one can do is to weigh up the potential harms that can occur and choose the course of action that produces the least harm.

To tell a client that a close relative no longer wishes to stay in contact with them is obviously hurtful. No matter how justifiable the reasons are, most people are likely to see it as a sign of rejection. To spare the feelings of a client, staff may continue to write letters but only pretend to post them and make excuses why the person can no longer visit. This strategy could be effective, providing the client never discovers that they are being deceived. However, as time passes and no replies to their letters are received, staff will have to tell more lies to account for the lack of news. Should the deceived client ever discover the truth, they are likely to experience not one harm but two: the original hurt of rejection by a former close relative, and the additional deception carried out by the care staff. In addition, their relationship with staff will be put in jeopardy. How will they be able to trust what staff say to them? Almost certainly they risk greater potential damage from the deception than from being told the truth.

If clients are suffering from a severe handicap, staff may feel that the chances of them discovering the deception are remote. Consequently, to spare them the hurt of rejection they may feel it serves their interests better to continue with the pretence of writing letters. However, if individuals are completely incapable of understanding that they are being deceived, it is unlikely that rejection will make much sense to them either. This calls into question the need to lie in the first place. It only serves to save staff from the difficult job of breaking unwelcome news.

The main objection to lying is that it erodes relationships. Consequently, lying or deliberately setting out to deceive, weakens any existing bonds of trust between carer and client.

Sometimes, ethical dilemmas arise when staff genuinely believe that a deception is in the best interests of clients. One of the most familiar examples of this is when a doctor prescribes a placebo to a patient. A placebo is a harmless substance given to a patient who is under the impression that he or she is taking a proper medicine.

The decision to use a placebo can be well-intentioned. It may be because a patient has already been given the maximum dosage of a pain-killing drug but continues to ask for more. A doctor might resort to using a placebo knowing that it is harmful to exceed the dose. If an injection of distilled water eases the patient's pain then the doctor is likely to feel justified in practising the deception. The strange thing about placebos is that if an individual expects them to work, they often do!

The administration of placebos is not usually likely to be a matter of concern to care staff, but it can serve as an example where deception might cause less harm to a client than a truthful explanation why they can be given no more painkillers.

It needs to be stressed that pain control is a complex subject and staff should always take it seriously. Pain is what the patient perceives it to be and not what a health professional thinks it is. Doctors and nurses must make every attempt to ensure a client does not suffer pain or, if that is impossible, at least to reduce the pain to tolerable levels.

 Action exercise 4.4 _____

Most people have told lies once in a while. From your own experiences identify occasions when you have been untruthful. Give examples of a lie which you thought was justifiable in the circumstances (and the reasons to justify it). Give examples of lies which on reflection you now feel were not justified.

Consent to deception

Deceiving individuals is not always unethical. Often people give their consent to be deceived. An interesting book or exciting film is a deception which most people are happy to experience. Actors and actresses are not acting unethically when they entertain us with fictional situations, or magicians when they practise illusions.

People can volunteer to be deceived in other ways. Sometimes a patient suffering from a terminal illness may say to a doctor 'If it is bad news then I don't want to be told about it'. Many doctors, hearing this, would willingly enter the deception and withhold the unwelcome details of the illness. Unfortunately, when some patients have wanted to be told the seriousness of their condition, doctors and nurses have also withheld the truth. Such deceptions are difficult to justify. The task of telling someone that they are going to die is not an easy one. However, withholding the truth from someone who wants to know it is sparing the feelings of the health professional rather than the patient.

There may be occasions when practising a deception is definitely in the interests of a client. An example of this is when an individual, through confusion or paranoia, refuses to take a prescribed medicine essential to their health. To safeguard the person's health, it might be necessary to administer the drug by deception, perhaps disguised in a drink or sandwich.

The times when deliberate deception is justifiable are so rare that staff should fully discuss the reasons why they think it is necessary. If an individual refuses life-saving medication, senior staff are likely to make an application to place the person under a section of the Mental Health Act. Therefore any deception that is necessary is legally permissible. If there is a reason to deceive clients, it should always be only after joint staff discussions, and as part of a recorded formal plan of care. It should never be because individual carers in their own interests, or on the spur of the moment, have decided to withhold the truth from clients.

 Case study _____

Mrs Shadwell is a 70-year-old lady admitted to a nursing care home about a year ago. She is a pleasant-natured lady, fairly quiet and 'not one to make a fuss'. Her married son visits her regularly and constantly complains about her care. According to him nothing is right – she is not getting enough food, she is dressed untidily, her clothes need washing etc. To an unbiased observer the complaints are clearly not justified. She receives first-class care and never complains directly to staff about anything. After her son's visit she appears embarrassed and apologises to staff for his conduct. Discuss this situation and possible reasons for the behaviour of both the client and her son. Also what actions, if any, do you think staff should take?

Summary of key points

- Effective communication is an important part of the relationship between client and carer.
- Staff must assist clients in overcoming barriers to communication.
- Staff require to be proficient in understanding and using non-verbal means of communication.
- Communicating by touch can be effective but clients' wishes need to be known and respected.
- 'Talking down' to clients devalues them and singles them out as being different.
- Self-advocacy is the practice of speaking out on one's own behalf to safeguard personal interests.
- Citizen advocacy is when an individual speaks on behalf of another person to secure their entitlements.
- Trust is necessary to the establishment of good relationships and effective communication.
- Staff should be truthful in their communications with clients or when acting as their spokesperson.
- Withholding the truth from clients may be justifiable on rare occasions, but only when agreed by others and when part of a formal plan of care.

Chapter 5
Privacy

Trust and privacy

The importance that trust plays in establishing a satisfying relationship with clients has already been mentioned. However, trust is not something that happens overnight, it takes time to build up. Unfortunately a thoughtless act can cause it to disappear in a flash.

Few people enjoy being gossiped about, or having their private affairs discussed in public. Like the rest of us, clients need to feel secure that what they say and do in confidence is not discussed with anyone else. If staff fail to keep the personal affairs of their clients confidential, they are guilty of a breach of trust. They are also failing to show respect. Privacy is a right which most people value highly, and respect for persons also involves respecting their rights.

In residential care there are many situations which call for privacy. Obvious examples are when clients require help in dressing, bathing or going to the lavatory. It is clearly impossible for clients to retain their dignity, if they have to undertake these personal intimate activities in public.

There are other occasions too, when staff should make efforts to respect the privacy of residents. From time to time everybody experiences moments when they want to be left alone. If anything, living with a number of other people probably increases the desire for occasional periods of solitude.

Part of a carer's role is to observe clients to make sure that they are safe. Observational skills are also necessary to judge a client's mood and state of mind. There is little point in engaging a client in an activity if they are not in the mood to participate. However, clients will need respite from being continuously watched. Most people welcome the opportunity to escape periodically to a quiet retreat, where no demands are made upon them. Carers have to strike a balance between observing clients and respecting their desire for solitude.

Each day it should be possible to allow clients the freedom to escape from prying eyes and unwanted interruptions, making sure that this is what they want, and that it is safe to leave them alone.

The need to be alone occasionally is quite normal, providing it is part of an individual's usual behaviour pattern. A sudden wish for long periods of isolation however, could be a sign that something is wrong, especially if previously a client enjoyed mixing with other people. Someone who sits permanently alone showing no desire for companionship, or retires to their room, could be suffering from depression, particularly if this behaviour is out of character. A client who suddenly becomes excessively secretive and furtive may be simply trying to obtain a little more privacy. On the other hand, they could be showing early signs of paranoia, and require medical attention.

Individuals vary tremendously in their need for privacy. Some want comparatively little, preferring instead to socialise with their fellows, while others are more introspective, requiring company only in small amounts. If this is their normal behaviour then their wishes should be respected. However, any sudden changes in a client's usual behaviour, *for no apparent reason*, should always be brought to the attention of senior staff.

Sexual expression

Expressing sexuality is an integral part of human activity. Most people quickly learn that its more intimate aspects require privacy, as public displays of sexual behaviour can be illegal, or simply embarrassing to passers-by. Clients living in residential care have the same sexual desires as the staff who look after them. Like them, they may want to express their sexuality, but unlike staff they often have fewer opportunities to do so in private.

The sexual needs of clients will vary as they do for everybody. In the case of some elderly residents, they may be mainly concerned in making the most of their appearance. They may want to be dressed in the right clothes, properly shaved or wearing their favourite make-up before putting in their first public appearance of the day. Care staff should be alert and sensitive to these wishes.

Some clients, even elderly ones, may have more physical sexual needs to consider. Comparatively few are likely to be living in an establishment where they can experience a full sexual relationship with a partner. If they are, then they will require privacy to enjoy their relationship.

Others, less fortunate, may find that their main release from sexual tension is by self-stimulation or masturbation. To express their sexuality, they require surroundings that can provide them with privacy. This may not be easy, particularly for clients who have to share bedrooms. Even if a bedroom is shared, it is possible to reserve it for single occupancy at least some times during the day.

Staff have to address these problems sensitively. It is unlikely that clients will openly discuss sexual matters and therefore carers should demonstrate thoughtfulness and tact in ensuring that clients have opportunities to be undisturbed at times.

Privacy also extends to the personal possessions of clients and to the lockers containing them. These should be out of bounds to staff. They could contain pictures or magazines that some might find offensive. Even if they are no more suggestive than some of the pin-up photographs seen daily in the tabloid press, clients may not want others to know of their interest in such items. As long as the controversial material is not illegal, and is kept in its owner's possession, it is not the duty of staff to act as censors.

Staff attitudes

Carers, because of the values they hold, are sometimes guilty of ignoring the sexual needs of their clients. They may forget that sexuality is not restricted only to the young and able-bodied. Like other members of the public, members of staff can be affected by media images, as well as by their own upbringing.

Without doubt the media plays an important part in fashioning public attitudes towards sex. Films, television and advertisements are constantly communicating a message that sex is for the young and the beautiful. In the artificial world of Hollywood, women sex symbols are invariably blonde, leggy, and curvaceous, while male 'hunks' are tall, muscular and good looking.

The huge amounts of money spent on cosmetics and beauty treatments, by both sexes, is evidence that these images do influence people even though most are aware that real life is very different from glossy pictures in magazines.

Most individuals do not have the features or figure to measure up to the popular image of 'sexiness' but despite this, regardless of their shape, size, physical appearance or age, people continue to have sexual desires. The feelings that they have can be just as intense as those felt by supposedly more glamorous beings.

 Action exercise 5.1 _____

Discuss to what extent you think that people are influenced by the media in the values that they hold regarding sexual behaviour. Do you think controversial subjects like homosexuality, prostitution, or AIDS are usually portrayed negatively or positively?

Many people, both in middle age and in later years, still want to express their sexuality. In some cases, the passionate emotions of youth may be less fervent, but nevertheless they still remain. Some individuals retain strong sexual desires well into old age. Neither physical disabilities nor mental impairment prevent individuals from possessing feelings of sexual desire.

The values that we hold about sex are often deeply ingrained because of our own upbringing. While some feel disgust at the thought of homosexuality, others are more accepting, even though they themselves may not be gay. Masturbation in any form, to some people, is a sinful activity, but for others, it may be the only way to satisfy their sexual feelings.

Care workers are also members of the public and many of the values they hold will be representative of the general population. Some of these values, we have seen, can be detrimental to the needs of people who make up the client group. Therefore staff should understand that their values, although important to them, should not be imposed upon clients in their care.

In practical terms, this means that a carer who disapproves of masturbation should nevertheless strive to provide privacy for a client who wishes to indulge in the activity. However, this does not mean that staff must not restrict sexual behaviour entirely; there may be good reasons for doing so.

A resident who tries to force unwelcome sexual attentions upon another must be prevented from doing so. Similarly, staff must stop clients from engaging in other unlawful sexual activities or inappropriate behaviours in public. However, this is very different from restricting a client's sexuality because the personal values of care staff do not approve of some forms of sexual expression.

Respecting privacy and maintaining confidentiality

Some clients will be extremely reluctant to discuss any aspect of sex. This may be especially noticeable with older people, who were brought up in less liberal times. The personal thoughts and feelings of people are worthy of respect. Staff should not ask intrusive questions concerning sexual attitudes or make risqué jokes to clients who dislike public expressions of sexuality. Nevertheless, clients who are reluctant to talk about sex may still experience strong desires. Like others, they must have opportunities to enjoy time on their own.

Clients can experience sexual feelings towards members of staff. Although rare, it sometimes does happen, particularly with younger clients, who may be immature or even confused about their own sexuality. If a member of staff suspects that a client is physically attracted to them, they should report their concerns to a senior member of staff. Misplaced feelings can be a potential source of distress for both client and carer alike. Later in this book we will discuss how accusations of abuse can jeopardise an individual's future. For now, it is enough to remember that the duty of staff is to protect clients and not to take advantage of them.

Just as some individuals are reluctant to discuss sexual matters, others are more than eager to do so. Some clients may even find it easier to discuss personal matters with staff than with friends or relatives. It is essential that any conversations of a personal nature between client and carer remain confidential, unless there are particularly pressing reasons to justify the breaking of a confidence.

Not all information passed from client to carer is confidential.

Most clients will acknowledge that it is in their own interests for certain information to be accessible to all staff. Comments regarding their current health status are commonly reported; so too is routine information regarding such things as sleeping patterns. These types of observational notes can help day staff, coming on duty, to understand why a client might be reluctant to get out of bed, or appears to be excessively sleepy during the daytime. A regular pattern of disturbed sleep can sometimes be a sign that someone is suffering from depression.

Records should be accurate and contain only relevant information. A client with epilepsy, for example, requires details concerning their fits to be entered on an appropriate chart. Information regarding the time, number and type of fit is invaluable to any doctor prescribing anti-convulsant drugs. As a result of the information, a doctor may have to prescribe a more effective drug, or alter the dosages of existing medication, especially if the record shows that fits are increasing in number or duration. Therefore, comments on seizure charts or records should be confined to describing the type of fit and when and where it occurred. With handwritten records they must be legible too. There is little point in recording information that nobody else can read.

In addition to general information, clients' records will also contain confidential material. They are likely to have details of family history and past illnesses. Consequently, it is important that confidential documents are kept in a secure place and not left lying around when not in use.

Organisations will vary in their policies and practices regarding confidentiality. In some establishments, staff will be among a select few who have access to certain information. Therefore, they will have more responsibilities regarding the safekeeping of information than other workers. However, every member of staff has a duty of confidentiality, regardless of whether they have access to records or not.

All employers should have policies regarding confidential material that they should make clear to their staff. Employees should comply with their particular employer's policies, and risk disciplinary action or dismissal if they fail to do so.

Increasingly, confidential records are being kept in electronic form on computers. Staff who have access to these records must be particularly vigilant regarding their security. If passwords are used to gain access to files, they should be kept confidential and not written down on scraps of paper for others to see. Also passwords should not be so obvious that they are easy to guess. It is not a good idea to use the date of one's own birthday or name of a favourite pet or pop star as a password.

Policies regarding confidentiality

A considerable amount of legislation exists which has implications for maintaining confidentiality. The Data Protection Act 1984, the Medical Act 1983 and the Access to Health Records Act 1990 are some typical examples. Many of the local policies drawn up by care establishments will include some of the major recommendations of these acts.

Employers therefore have a duty to ensure that staff are aware of the implications of any legislation that is relevant to their particular role. In turn, staff have a duty to follow the statutory requirements of legislation and the policies of their employer.

When new laws are passed and existing ones updated, employers need to ensure that staff receive ongoing training. Breaches of confidentiality can have serious repercussions and ignorance of the law is not an excuse. Individuals cannot escape responsibility if they make unintentional disclosures by claiming a lack of knowledge. It is thus in the staff's own interests to be aware of the implications of any new or current regulations.

Whether they have access to records or not, care staff have to be particularly careful about disclosing information unintentionally. Colleagues sometimes travel home together from work by public transport and can easily get into the habit of talking about the day's events at work. The danger with such conversations is that confidential matters concerning clients can be overheard by other passengers. Even if staff refrain from breaching confidentiality themselves, they must not encourage others to do so, by inviting them to gossip about particular clients.

Action exercise 5.2

Values clarification:

Answer the questions and then compare and discuss your answers with the rest of the group.

1. How would you personally feel if information you had given in confidence was disclosed without your permission?
2. Can you think of an instance when it might be justifiable for someone to disclose information you had given them in confidence? If so – provide examples.
3. Have you ever broken a confidence without justification? If so describe the occasion.
4. Do you ever read or pass on 'gossip' and what are your feelings about this?

Caution has to be exercised when asked for information about clients on the telephone. There will be a policy regarding this and it should be rigorously followed. If no policy exists, then staff should not reveal any personal information about clients without proof of the caller's identity. Anyone can claim to be a relative or social worker on the telephone. In addition, callers should make it clear why they are seeking certain information. A journalist writing an article on the health problems of elderly people might feel it justifiable to ask for specific information over the telephone. However, it may require the approval of senior staff to give out particular information, and the best response in these types of situations is to ask the caller to put the request in writing to the most senior member of staff.

On occasions, clients or relatives may be asked to provide a considerable amount of personal information, especially when clients are first admitted. When this happens, it should be explained in a sensitive manner, that other staff will have access to some of the information. At the same time, any policies regarding the safekeeping of records should be outlined, so that both clients and relatives are satisfied that a confidential environment prevails.

If clients or their advocates express reluctance about information being passed on, their anxieties should be taken seriously and sufficient time made available to discuss their concerns. Sometimes, it is possible to guarantee that access to information is selective. This means that some staff will have access to the information but not others. However, it is essential for some information to be available to all carers.

If a client is a severe diabetic, for instance, it is in their own interests that all staff are aware of this. A person who falls into a diabetic coma can die. Managers of a residential home would almost certainly face charges of negligence if they deliberately prevented staff from knowing such important information about a client. Therefore, in a situation like this, it would not be possible to agree to any request to withhold information from some members of staff. This fact would need to be explained diplomatically to clients or their relatives. The explanation should make clear that all staff who have access to information also have a duty of confidentiality. Even when it is possible to restrict access to records, there may be times when it is justifiable to divulge the confidential information contained within them.

Justifiable disclosures

Sometimes it is necessary to inform staff, who do not usually have access to records, that a client's condition is causing concern. If a client becomes seriously depressed and confides to a carer that they are contemplating suicide, then everyone involved in that client's care must be told of the situation, whether or not they usually have access to records. A client might see such a revelation as a breach of trust. However, the potential harm resulting from disclosure is less serious than allowing a mentally ill patient to kill him- or herself. It is possible in time for a client to re-establish a trusting relationship, even if it is with a different carer. However, if a suicide attempt is successful, the client has no further opportunities to relate to anyone.

Breaches of confidentiality can also be justifiable if they are in the public interest. A disturbed client who tells a member of staff that they have an urge to set fire to the building is clearly dangerous; to themselves as well as to others. Consequently, all staff should be aware of the potential threat – whether or not the person really intends to carry it out.

It is also justifiable to disclose confidential information, if directed to do so by a magistrate or a judge. Staff, like other members of the public, are answerable to the law. They have no special privilege that allows them to ignore an order of a court. Indeed, a refusal to divulge information can lead to an individual being charged with contempt of court and facing a fine or imprisonment.

If staff come into possession of information regarding illegal activities by others, they need to be careful not to make promises concerning confidentiality, which they may be unable to keep. If a client admits to a member of staff that they are involved in drug dealing or shoplifting, for instance, staff may have no choice but to report the facts to a senior manager. Failure to do this could be seen as condoning criminal activity and even lead to accusations of being an accomplice.

If it becomes necessary to disclose confidential information, staff should first inform clients of their intentions and the reasons why disclosure is necessary. If possible, clients should be persuaded to reveal the information themselves to an appropriate person. If they refuse to do so, staff should pass on the information and then inform the client of what they have done.

 Action exercise 5.3

Values clarification:

Answer the questions and then discuss your answers with the rest of the group.

1. Do care staff have a right to know if one of their clients has AIDS or is HIV positive? Explain your reasons.
2. Should clients have similar rights regarding the health status of their carers? Explain your reasons.
3. Do you think that someone working as a paid professional (care worker, nurse, doctor, social worker, solicitor etc.) has a greater responsibility to maintain confidentiality than a friend or member of the public? Please give reasons.
4. A colleague who is a relative (or close friend) of a long-serving member of staff informs you that the individual has a serious drink problem. She also thinks that it is affecting the person's work and putting clients at risk. She implores you not to reveal that she is the source of this information as it will damage her relationship with the person. What action (if any) do you take?

Dilemmas of confidentiality

Normally, close friends or family who regularly visit or telephone a client, expect to be kept informed of their relative's progress. Part of a care worker's duties involves liaising with relatives and, if possible, getting them to participate in the care of clients. There might be occasions, however, when a resident requests that certain information is not passed on – even to a close relative.

This can cause difficulties for staff who, over the years, may have built up a strong relationship with visiting relatives, especially if they are put into a position where they have to tell lies. A client, for instance, who develops a serious health problem may not want the news passed on to a visiting son or daughter. Perhaps they do not want to cause their grown-up children any additional worries, or they are afraid of becoming an object of pity and would prefer to be treated normally. Whatever the reasons, if the relative enquires about the client's health, it poses problems for staff. To answer truthfully betrays the client by revealing what they want kept confidential. The alternative is almost as bad. For lying to the relative is also a betrayal of trust, albeit to a different person.

Apart from any ethical dilemmas that staff might face, there are other issues to consider. Relatives will feel aggrieved if they are not kept informed about the health of a loved one, especially if the client becomes suddenly ill and dies, or if the relatives are contributing towards the costs of care.

There are limits to the actions that care staff may undertake in carrying out their role. Firstly, staff should not make a decision to deliberately lie to clients or to relatives. Secondly, staff should not be put into a position where they have no other choice but to lie. Thirdly, nursing home policies should make it clear to carers which senior member of staff to go to for advice and support when it is needed.

A client who says something in confidence to one carer may, without the carer's knowledge, repeat the information to another member of staff. If, as in the earlier example, it was a request not to pass on information concerning their health to a relative, problems can arise if staff act beyond the limits of their role. One carer might decide that the next-of-kin should be kept informed of the client's deteriorating health, while a second carer might decide that it is better to withhold the truth from relatives. In time the truth will be discovered, and both clients and relatives are likely to feel betrayed at being deceived. The relationship between fellow workers may also suffer, if each blames the other for the resulting chaos.

The prime responsibility of a care establishment is towards its clients. However, it also has some responsibilities towards other people, like relatives and next-of-kin. Staff should always be able to go to an experienced manager for guidance and support, when conflicts arise between competing interests, particularly where matters of privacy and confidentiality are concerned. If staff are uncertain what to do, they should not commit themselves to a promise of confidentiality, at least until they have had an opportunity to talk to their manager.

Limits to privacy

Even in our everyday lives there are limits to privacy. Just as computers have become capable of storing huge amounts of information, increasingly people are having to reveal more about themselves, for example when opening a bank account, applying for a job or taking out a mortgage on a house.

It is difficult to go shopping anywhere these days without video cameras watching us. However, while being under constant surveillance is an intrusion of privacy, most people gladly accept the spying cameras in exchange for the extra security they provide.

One of the few places left where people are able to retain their privacy is where they live. At home people can lock their front door, draw the curtains and retire from public view. They can have private conversations with partners, secure in the knowledge that they will not be overheard. When alone, they can please themselves what they do – even indulge in behaviour which other people might find offensive.

Care staff should strive to provide the same levels of privacy for clients living in a residential home. Inevitably there will be times when they will fail. Residential homes usually contain more people than a normal house which poses practical problems. Residents have to be kept under close observation, because their physical or mental conditions can make them vulnerable to accidents. Nevertheless, staff should at least strive to provide as much privacy for clients as they would enjoy if living at home.

 Case study _____

Sophie is an 18-year-old Down's Syndrome girl who comes into respite care at weekends. She is a pleasant well behaved young lady but staff find that she is prone to fantasising and exaggerating at times. She is particularly attached to Louise, one of the care staff. One day, she tells Louise that when she is at home her 17-year-old brother Alex does 'naughty things' with her. According to Sophie, when their parents are out, Alex persuades her to join him in undressing and they play 'touching' games together. She says although she loves Alex, she feels 'dirty' afterwards. She implores Louise to keep this information a secret as she doesn't want to get Alex into trouble. Discuss what you think Louise should do in these circumstances.

Summary of key points

- Respect for persons involves respecting their rights of privacy.
- If a need for privacy suddenly becomes overwhelming it could be a sign that something is wrong.
- Clients living in residential care have sexual needs in the same way as the staff who look after them.
- It is important that staff recognise that their own values regarding sexuality should not be imposed upon clients.
- Staff have a duty to ensure that any information they receive in confidence should not be revealed to others, except in extremely rare circumstances.
- Records should be accurate, legible and contain only relevant information.
- Confidential records should be kept in a secure place and not be left lying around when not in use.
- Policies regarding confidentiality will have to take account of legislation such as the Data Protection Act 1984, the Medical Act 1983 and the Access to Health Records Act 1990.
- It should be explained to clients, in an appropriate way, that other members of staff will have access to some of their personal information.

- It is justifiable to divulge confidential information if it is to protect the interests of a client or members of the public or by order of a court official.
- There are limits to the actions that staff may take in carrying out their role. If they are uncertain what to do, they should not commit themselves to a promise of confidentiality until they have spoken to senior staff.
- There are limits to confidentiality and to privacy in everyone's life, but staff should strive to provide as much privacy for clients as possible.

Chapter 6
Discrimination

Discrimination and equality

Treating clients fairly is an essential part of the duties of a care worker. Clients should experience neither unfair discrimination nor undue favouritism. Although not all clients will receive equal treatment, they should all receive treatment that is fair. If clients have special needs, it is sometimes justifiable to treat them in different ways in order for them to satisfy those needs.

Good reasons exist to explain why some clients will have special requirements. For example, because one resident may require a soft diet, it does not mean that all clients have the same requirement. Treating people differently is not in itself wrong. This kind of discrimination is acceptable and indeed necessary to fulfil any special needs.

Discrimination is often defined as the power of observing differences accurately, or of making exact distinctions and, as such, it is an essential part of our daily life. For instance, the ability to discriminate between colours when approaching traffic lights is an important part of our survival skills. However, to discriminate between people on the basis of a prejudiced or unfair perspective is both wrong and repugnant.

Everyone has a right to fair treatment. Consequently, there can be no room for bias or prejudice in the way that staff care for their clients. Unfair discrimination disadvantages individuals, because it deprives them of opportunities that others take for granted. It usually arises, not from rational thinking, but from ignorance and a mixture of powerful emotions such as fear, jealousy or hatred.

Apathy and thoughtlessness can also be responsible for prejudiced viewpoints. Sometimes, individuals merely take on board the attitudes of other influential people, without analysing or examining them too closely. The crime that discrimination commits is not that it treats people unequally, but that it treats them unfairly.

Types of discrimination

Discrimination appears in many forms. The types that attract the most publicity are usually those that focus upon an individual's racial, religious, or sexual characteristics. There are many other types of discrimination, some more obvious than others.

One that is unfortunately growing, as the policy of care in the community develops, is 'Not In My Back Yard', or NIMBY. This describes a situation when the public gives general approval to a policy – providing it takes place somewhere else!

The intention to resettle inmates with learning disabilities from institutions into houses in the community is a social policy that apparently attracts national support. The public's enthusiasm for the resettlement plans often disappears however, if they learn that a house within their own neighbourhood is to provide a new home for the former inmates. The reasons given why the resettlement house should be in a different neighbourhood are not always convincing. According to some, the market value of their own property will fall; others worry that street parking may become a problem, because of cars belonging to staff working in the new facility. These reasons often fail to stand up to close scrutiny. The majority of people with learning disabilities already live in the community, and property values do not plummet when they move house. Furthermore, it is unlikely that many more than two or three staff will be on duty at any one time, therefore parking problems will be no worse than those caused by many other families moving into the area.

This type of discrimination is subtle. Protesters are not saying that people with learning difficulties should not live in the community. They are even claiming to be sympathetic to the idea, pointing out that they are not against the policy itself – only its place of implementation. Most of the arguments that protesters make, if valid, would apply equally to other neighbourhoods. The protests they make are usually motivated more from self-interest than from malice. Nevertheless, they are no less damaging.

It is not only people with learning disabilities who face such prejudice. Individuals with a mental illness often face similar discrimination, especially if plans to open a new day clinic or hostel locally are in progress. Proposed new homes for the elderly have also been objected to on various grounds. The reasons given are rarely based on rational arguments.

Many employers are reluctant to offer jobs to people who have a history of mental illness, even if they are currently in good health and have been so for a number of years. Employers also frequently discriminate against older job seekers. The cut-off age for many jobs can be as low as 40 years old. Consequently, people in their late fifties or early sixties stand little chance of obtaining full-time employment.

Care staff should understand the potentially damaging effects that discrimination can have upon individuals, and recognise it when it occurs. For the sake of their clients, they must be aware of the causes of discrimination and how to reduce the chances of it happening in their own working environment.

Sources of prejudice

Prejudice is an opinion or attitude formed beforehand, and it is usually unfavourable and based on inadequate facts. It fuels the hatred that precedes acts of unfair discrimination. Carried to an excess, prejudice develops into a belief system that is incapable of change, despite any new evidence to the contrary.

In the first half of the century much popular art, with the notable exception of jazz, was a major source of racial prejudice and discrimination. Many books portrayed characters using words like 'nigger' or 'chinks' to describe members of different ethnic groups. Black actors were cast in roles depicting menial jobs such as janitors or butlers, while white artists invariably played the lead in films and plays. Whether it was Tarzan fighting off hordes of hostile natives, or cowboys defending women and children from Red Indian savages, heroes were always white and villains were any colour but white.

During this period, few ordinary people took holidays abroad. Immigrants arriving from other countries were comparatively few.

Most of the knowledge that people had about other cultures was derived from the stereotypes of popular entertainment. About the same time that Hollywood was at its most influential, a number of extreme organisations sprang up in Europe, some believing that their own culture was superior to that of others. This belief led to widespread acts of discrimination. In Germany this was particularly evident in the way that Jews and some other groups were treated.

However, the messages of cultural intolerance given out by these countries had comparatively little effect on people's attitudes in this country and the United States, in comparison with the negative cultural influences of popular entertainment. It was hardly surprising, therefore, that people developed a biased view of those individuals who were constantly being portrayed as inferior or evil.

Thankfully, things have improved. Black actors now take leading roles in films, and the parts they play can be prestigious ones. The language of popular fiction no longer contains words with offensive racial overtones.

However, the formative years of many older people were influenced by negative images of race and colour. Consequently, some may still retain feelings of prejudice – even hatred – and clients can be active sources of discrimination. Relatives, visitors and other care staff are also capable of prejudice. Discrimination is by no means unique to the older generation. Sadly, the recent rise in pro-Nazi organisations, many of which have a largely youthful membership, is living testament to this fact.

 Action exercise 6.1 _____

From personal experience, identify a situation in which you witnessed or experienced discrimination and describe how you felt at the time. Alternatively, identify an occasion when you felt prejudiced towards an individual or group and explain what your present feelings are towards the individual(s).

There are various degrees of prejudice. It can sometimes be positive as well as negative and to some extent it exists in everybody. It might not necessarily be a bigoted hatred, but more a display of favouritism towards certain other individuals or groups. We are all guilty, at times, of acting in a way that is not impartial.

Most people usually show some positive bias towards their friends or family. They are more likely to offer them help or support than they would a comparative stranger. Individuals are also more likely to see themselves in a complimentary light. Few motorists, for instance, consider themselves to be bad drivers. It is nearly always the other driver who is careless and at fault.

It is almost impossible to be totally free from some form of self-deception and most reasonable persons, on reflection, will probably admit to being biased in some areas of their life. After all, it is hardly surprising that people usually treat friends better than strangers. Consequently, most people accept favouritism as an inescapable form of prejudice, at least when it concerns close friends and loved ones.

Residential care staff, however, are in a different position to members of the general public. The relationship they have with clients is already unequal in terms of power, and if they are to start dispensing special favours to some clients, but not others, the imbalance in power will increase even further. It must be remembered too, that showing favouritism to some clients can only be at the expense of discriminating unfairly against others.

Acting impartially

One of the most common ways in which staff discriminate against clients is by avoiding them. This was highlighted in Chapter 3 where a research study was discussed on nurses' attitudes towards unpopular patients. It is impossible to view everyone we meet with the same affection. Care staff are no different from everybody else in this circumstance.

Care staff will relate to some people more warmly than others, some they will have no strong feelings about either way, others they may view with some distaste. These feelings are normal and carers should not feel guilty simply because they experience them. Nevertheless, although it may be impossible to stop experiencing certain emotions, individuals can control their feelings. If they are unable to do so, then they are likely to be working in the wrong job.

We do not have to act upon the emotions that we feel, nor, if we are in a position of responsibility, is it justifiable to do so. Instead, staff have to adopt a professional approach to their clients. This involves carrying out duties according to the needs of the client and not the carer. A professional approach means that staff do not become too emotionally entangled with individual clients. This does not mean that they have to be aloof and distant, or cold and unapproachable. It is still possible to display a friendly or caring manner while maintaining limits to the degree of intimacy entering a relationship.

Carers should aim to be even handed in their treatment of clients. They should display neither favouritism to some, nor hostility to others. Above all, they have to be in control of their own emotions to ensure that they do not discriminate unfairly against some clients.

It is also important for carers to identify their own values and possible prejudices towards certain groups. For unless they can recognise areas of bias in their own attitudes they will be unable to deal with them. A good manager will try to promote an atmosphere where staff feel confident to approach them for support in coming to terms with anxieties or negative emotions. Staff may have to make an extra effort to understand the sensitivities of others and learn how to relate to them better.

Staff discrimination

Avoiding clients is one possible form of staff discrimination. There are unfortunately many others. A resident who has regular bouts of incontinence can be made to feel dirty, even disgusting by the attitudes and behaviour of care staff. Whether unintentionally or not, a carer's body language can send strong messages of hostility to a client. Feelings of repugnance are sometimes unwittingly expressed by the brusque manner in which staff attend to the cleaning up and changing of soiled clothes of incontinent clients. There have been occasions when members of staff have deliberately discriminated against incontinent clients. They feel these clients are intentionally 'dirty' and punish them by making them wait long periods before attending to their needs. Some even compound this neglect with verbal abuse, publicly criticising the unfortunate individual for their condition. In the next chapter we will look in more detail at examples of ill treatment.

The effects of discriminating unfairly against clients can be far-reaching. Other clients, grateful not to be the targets of adverse comments themselves, may mimic the prejudiced attitudes of the staff in order to demonstrate 'whose side they are on'. If incontinent clients are publicly accused by staff of being 'dirty,' then their peers, to curry staff favour, may join the chorus of disapproval to show that they are 'clean'.

It is not only incontinent clients who are subject to animosity; those who have episodes of confusion can also suffer. A client who is forgetful might wander around with items of clothing missing, possibly wearing odd shoes or even ones that are on the wrong feet. If staff make unthinking comments, or laugh openly at the person's behaviour, it could be a trigger for other clients to do the same. People in a vulnerable position are only too pleased not to become scapegoats themselves, and one way of achieving this is to ensure that someone else fulfils that role.

Care staff should not only refrain from unfair discrimination themselves but they should also encourage others to do the same. If a colleague or client is guilty of making inappropriate prejudicial comments, it should be pointed out that this practice is unacceptable. It should also be explained to the offender the possible damaging consequences of their discriminatory words or actions.

If the establishment has a written anti-discrimination policy, staff who contravene it should receive a reminder of its existence. However, before reproaching others, staff must be confident that their own standards of fairness are above reproach. They need to examine their own consciences to make sure that they themselves are not guilty of discriminating unfairly against others, particularly clients with whom they have little in common.

If staff experience problems relating to a 'difficult' client, they should seek the advice of a senior member of staff, even if it means admitting that they do not like the person and find it hard to care for them.

If staff normally carry out their duties proficiently, managers will probably welcome an honest approach for support. From their viewpoint, it is better to avoid potential problems than to have to resolve them later. It might be possible for the carer to work with other clients, or work in close cooperation with another colleague while attending to the client. It may be that they have to get to know the client better, or simply have an opportunity to talk to someone else about their feelings.

If a person approaches a member of staff to complain about unfair discrimination they should receive cooperation and support. Dealing with complaints will be looked at in more detail later. However, staff should take complaints seriously whether made by clients, colleagues or visitors. For instance, if someone complains to a carer about a colleague's alleged inappropriate comments, it is not acceptable to attempt to dismiss them as 'a bit of fun' or by suggesting that the person complaining is being 'oversensitive'.

Effects of ignorance and class

There are almost as many reasons for discrimination as there are groups who are discriminated against. As stated previously, ignorance is often a major factor. In recent years this has been evident in the public perception of people who are HIV positive. Employers have not always been sympathetic. Many sufferers have lost their jobs once news of their condition became known, others have been unable to get a mortgage or life insurance. HIV positive children have even been excluded from attending schools or playing with others.

The public's fear of AIDS in the early days was largely due to ignorance. In recent years, however, people have generally become more knowledgeable about the condition. This has helped reduce some of the worst cases of discrimination, although by no means all.

Children born with the condition, or those who become HIV positive as a result of a blood transfusion, do attract sympathy. However those who acquire the condition through sexual intercourse, or drug abuse, obtain little compassion. Because of the lifestyle they lead, victims are often blamed for bringing the condition upon themselves – and for passing it on to others. The general discrimination that prevails against homosexuality does not help matters. Frequently, people still see AIDS as a disease only relevant to a minority group.

As with so many of our beliefs, childhood influences are often a powerful factor in the process of discrimination. Working class children growing up on a council estate will meet and mingle with friends and peers from the same background. They will attend the same schools and probably share many of the same leisure interests. The people they meet most easily will share the same environment. They are also the ones with whom they are most likely to marry and set up home.

Similarly, children born to upper middle class parents will share common experiences and backgrounds, although very different ones. These may include a nanny in their formative years and later being educated as a boarder at a public or finishing school.

Given these influences it is not surprising that class differences can give rise to feelings of prejudice, with one group seeing the other as either 'posh' or 'common', depending upon their respective viewpoints. To some extent this is an oversimplification. People do cross over class barriers, perhaps through marriage or by career moves. Not everybody in one social class dislikes or discriminates against people from another. Nevertheless, the people we mix with in our formative years, including parents or guardians, exert a powerful influence upon us.

Victim blaming

AIDS is not the only condition for which people are blamed for bringing upon themselves. In recent years, this country has seen the promotion of an enterprise culture designed to encourage people to depend more upon their own efforts and increasingly less upon government help. In the United States this philosophy has been in existence from the earliest pioneering days.

The attitudes which people have towards self-help vary according to personal characteristics as well as political beliefs. Often individuals who are unable to help themselves attract less public sympathy than those who demonstrate the ability to control their lives. Instead, they are blamed for their perceived shortcomings and often discriminated against as well.

Insurance companies already charge higher premiums to insure people who are heavy smokers or overweight. Employers too, are increasingly reluctant to employ people they see as a health risk. Some argue that individuals should be more responsible for personal fitness and adopt a healthier lifestyle. They point out that a failure to do so increases the overheads of firms employing unhealthy workers, as well as escalating NHS costs.

These arguments have some merit, but they often fail to distinguish between people's circumstances. A poorly educated young mother, living on income support in a high-rise tower block, and trying to cope with the demands of young children, has intense pressures in her daily life. The withdrawal symptoms associated with giving up smoking could lead to irritability provoking bouts of ill temper against her children. Her home cannot offer the same comfort that tobacco provides.

The stresses that a middle class suburban housewife face by comparison are significantly less. She is in a better position to seek support and advice in breaking the smoking habit. She can probably also afford some alternative pastime to replace her habit, such as joining a health and fitness club, or simply rewarding herself by putting the money saved from smoking towards a holiday.

It is easy to blame people for their shortcomings and to discriminate unfairly against them. Care staff must avoid this particular trap. Although both smoking and obesity are proven dangers to well-being, the role of care staff is not to act as health police. Their duty is to respect the autonomy of clients.

If clients wish to continue to smoke, regardless of the health risks, then they should be allowed to do so. However, they cannot smoke whenever and wherever they want, for there will be other non-smoking clients to consider. Instead, there should be a smoking area available, unless the home has a policy of non-smoking, and this was pointed out to the client prior to admission. If, however, they were originally admitted as a smoker, it is discriminatory not to allow them to continue, providing they keep to the rules or policies of the establishment.

 Action exercise 6.2 _____

Group discussion:

Do you think that, at times, people by their behaviour or lifestyle almost invite others to discriminate against them? If so, does this mean that there can be some occasions when discrimination can be excused or justified?

The same philosophy should apply to dieting. There are many instances where staff in long stay institutions have put inmates on diets to lose surplus pounds, often without any consultation with the client or their relatives. To make such decisions without client consent is discriminatory and unjustifiably paternalistic, especially if, as sometimes happens, the staff responsible are themselves overweight.

Carers have every right to point out to their clients that certain forms of behaviour are unhealthy. Part of their duties is to assist clients in maintaining optimum health. However, once they have done this they should not continue to nag, unless a client's behaviour places him or herself at *serious* risk of harm.

Sometimes, clients may not be fully rational. For instance, a resident who refuses to stick to a diabetic diet could lapse into a coma and die. In this case, common sense must prevail. If care staff are in any doubt about what to do in certain circumstances, they should *always* seek help from senior staff.

Preventing discrimination

At times, clients will discriminate against each other. Everyone has irritating habits or behaviours which annoy other people, and when individuals are living together in a small community, petty irritations can easily become magnified into full-scale provocations.

Some clients may be in the habit of talking to themselves loudly. Others may have hallucinations that spark off imaginary threats causing them to shout out in fear or anger. Noise can be disturbing and the unfortunate client can find themselves being reproached by peers. Once a resident gains a reputation for disruption, the possibility increases that remaining clients will exclude him or her from their circle of friendship.

In situations such as these, the role of the care worker is to protect the confused person from victimisation. By their own attitudes and behaviour, staff should set an appropriate example for the remaining clients to follow. This includes making it clear that it is unacceptable to make discriminatory remarks about other people. It is also part of their role to help resolve conflicts when they arise. If some individuals are shouting abuse at a disturbed resident, it is not only discriminatory, but it adds to the general noise and disruption, without providing any solution to the underlying problem.

Relatives and clients can be the focus of discrimination, especially if they attract a reputation among staff for being 'awkward'. Visitors are right to point out when the care of a relative falls below standard. Even in the best run homes mistakes can happen and sometimes things get overlooked. Providing staff deal with complaints speedily and offer a sincere apology, most people will be satisfied. Occasionally, however, this is not the case. Sometimes, it is possible to meet visitors who seem to be hypercritical about every aspect of care, even when it is of the highest quality.

The reasons for this type of behaviour can vary. Relatives may feel guilty that they were unable to cope with caring for the client and have had to hand over their responsibilities to paid staff. The resulting resentment may then be directed against all those involved in caring for the individual. Alternatively, they may believe that constant complaining 'keeps staff on their toes' and guarantees their relative first-class care. On the other hand, they may simply be awkward people who get some sort of enjoyment from perpetual fault finding. Invariably, staff do not look forward to the arrival of such visitors. When they appear, they sometimes try to avoid them, hoping that a luckless colleague will have to welcome them instead. Although an understandable reaction, this is not a professional way for staff to behave. Avoiding uncomfortable situations does nothing to resolve them. The discrimination that is directed towards the visitors also affects the relevant client. If staff are avoiding relatives, they are avoiding the people they care for too.

If a client is aware of staff resentment against their visitors it can place them in a difficult position and they can be pulled by conflicting loyalties, trying to please both carers and family. This is why staff must act in a professional way and interact with difficult relatives in the same way that they do with difficult clients.

 Action exercise 6.3 _____

What policies or legislation exist to promote anti-discriminatory practices and to which groups in society do they apply? Discuss any advantages or disadvantages they may have in reducing discrimination and what more, if anything, can be done by legislation to reduce discrimination.

Working as a team

Members of staff have a responsibility to set new employees acceptable standards to follow. If the normal pattern of behaviour is to treat clients fairly, then new staff are likely to adopt the same philosophy. Individuals with prejudice against people of a different culture are unlikely to broadcast their opinions, if the environment they work in is intolerant of discriminatory behaviour.

Care workers joining an existing team of staff will hope to become part of the group as quickly as possible. Usually, they will copy the group's standards of behaviour to win approval and gain acceptance. If the team view unfair discrimination as unacceptable in the provision of care, there is a likelihood that, to begin with, the new member will reflect the same attitudes.

In time, differences can arise in a team and, if they do, the resulting disharmony is usually detrimental to client care. Conflicts among staff can lead to divisions within the team. This can happen through misunderstandings between staff working on different shifts or even on the same shift.

Usually each group starts blaming the other for perceived inadequacies. Night staff may feel that carers working on days are leaving too much work for staff coming on duty, or vice versa. Once a group perceives another as being lazy, there is a risk that the conflict arising will lead to discrimination against clients. For example, a client who becomes incontinent during the last hour of a working shift might be left unattended for the next shift to deal with.

It is all too easy for clients to become pawns when staff battle among themselves and it is therefore vital that staff work in harmony. Differences when they arise have to be resolved. A cycle of petty squabbling between factions risks clients being discriminated against unfairly. It also presents an unsavoury spectacle to clients, if they witness care staff quarrelling among themselves.

Respect, risk and restrictions

Individuals can influence other people's perceptions of them by their own actions and behaviour. A person's appearance and the way that they behave sends out messages to others which can be mis-interpreted. A carer who hates formality may dress casually and be in the habit of addressing people in a relatively intimate manner – even comparative strangers.

These attempts to promote a free and easy manner in interactions with others can be misconstrued as showing a lack of respect. Clients who equate formality with politeness could perceive themselves as being treated rudely, especially if carers adopt different behaviour patterns with other people.

If staff act deferentially to visitors and senior colleagues but casually and offhand to clients, they are demonstrating a lack of regard for those in their care. Treating people differently for no justifiable reason is discriminatory.

Unintentional discrimination is just as damaging as deliberate discrimination, therefore staff should be aware of the possible effects of their behaviour on other people. Thoughtlessness on the part of a carer can provoke resentment by a client. If they are asked a question by a client which they are unable to answer, it should be referred to someone who can make an appropriate response.

A resident with a chronic health condition for example, may seek reassurance or information about their condition. It is unacceptable to brush such queries aside, as sometimes happens, with mean-ingless comments meant to reassure. Telling a client 'not to worry, you are looking fine' is patronising, as well as being unethical if the carer is ignorant of a client's real condition.

In such circumstances staff have to make clear to the client that they do not have the information that is being requested. To pretend otherwise is practising a deceit. However, they should also reassure the client that they will communicate the request for information to a senior member of staff who may be in a better position to answer their query.

People have a right to accurate information. Most individuals seeking information about their own health would feel angry if their GP ignored their questions. The chances of discrimination occurring are slight, when people treat others in the same way that they like to be treated themselves.

Although people have a right to information, they also have a right not to have it thrust at them. Not everyone wants to hear the details of a poor prognosis. If a client clearly does not wish to hear bad news concerning a serious health problem then that wish should be respected.

Conflicts can arise if a client requests details of their state of health and a relative does not think it appropriate for the person to be fully informed about their condition, especially if the news is likely to upset them. In these situations, senior staff, and others, have to be involved in deciding the best course of action. The views of relatives are always important and they should not be unduly distressed, but the interests of clients must always be the first concern of staff. Withholding information can only be justified if it causes clients less harm than divulging it.

Sometimes carers, even with the best of intentions, can act unfairly. They can become overprotective to clients if they think they are particularly vulnerable. For instance, they may place severe restrictions on the liberty of clients with epilepsy, through a misguided fear for their safety. However treating everyone suffering from epilepsy in an overprotective manner is itself discriminatory.

Some clients with epilepsy will have a few well-controlled seizures occasionally throughout the year. By contrast, others can have major fits each week which require urgent treatment, especially if they are prone to lapsing into the life threatening condition of *status epilepticus*. There are different forms of epilepsy and people are affected in different ways. Some receive mental warnings of an approaching fit, while others are less fortunate and their seizures commence suddenly and unexpectedly. Due to the differences in the types of fits and their severity, it is necessary to treat individuals differently. While carers must ensure that no clients are exposed to unnecessary dangers, there are times when acceptable risks can be taken to ensure a better quality of life for some clients.

Epilepsy invariably has an effect on the activities of daily living. A person with epilepsy who has a fit while bathing risks losing consciousness and drowning. Consequently, they require someone to be in close attendance while they bathe, which places severe restrictions upon their privacy. A client who experiences major fits on a regular basis must have a carer in the same room with them while bathing. However, it might be possible to offer more privacy to a client who experiences minor fits occasionally, and who also receives advance warnings of them. Someone who suffers only minor fits might only need a member of staff to be outside the bathroom with the door ajar. However, the decision to adopt this approach cannot be made by any individual member of staff; it would have to be part of a written care plan sanctioned by the approval of medical staff or senior managers, after discussions with the client and his or her relatives.

Nevertheless, the illustration serves to underline the importance of treating clients according to their needs. To place the same restrictions on everyone with a diagnosis of epilepsy, without assessing the severity of their condition, is discriminatory. The same holds true for clients who are diabetic or who suffer from bouts of confused behaviour or other debilitating conditions. Each case must be decided on its merits, otherwise the stereotypes associated with the particular condition invite discrimination.

 Case study _____

Mrs Jones regularly visits her 80-year-old mother who is a resident at the home where you work. She is generally appreciative of the way that staff look after her mother but constantly finds fault with Ethel, the only black carer currently employed. Mrs Jones claims that Ethel doesn't talk to her mother 'nicely' and that her mother is frightened of her. Nobody else has complained about Ethel, who is generally popular with everyone and considered to provide a good standard of care to all clients. How would you deal with this situation?

Summary of key points

- Everyone requires to be treated fairly. There is no room for bias in the way that staff look after their clients.
- The crime that discrimination commits, is not that it treats people unequally, but that it treats them unfairly.
- Care staff need to understand the potentially damaging effects that discrimination can have upon individuals.

- To some degree, prejudice exists in everybody. Everyone can be guilty at times of acting in a way that is not impartial.
- Care staff are no different from anybody else. There will be some people to whom they relate more warmly than others.
- Staff should adopt a professional approach, not getting too emotionally involved and aiming to be even-handed in their treatment of clients.
- It is unacceptable for staff to discriminate against a client's unhealthy lifestyle especially if they themselves are indulging in similar behaviours.
- If a colleague or client is guilty of making inappropriate pre-judicial comments, it should be pointed out that it is a practice which is unacceptable.
- If staff experience problems relating to a client, they should seek the advice of a senior member of staff.
- Carers should refer client's questions that they cannot answer to an appropriate member of the care team.
- Even with the best of intentions, carers can sometimes act unfairly by becoming overprotective to clients they view as being particularly vulnerable.
- The greatest contribution staff can make to promoting anti-discriminatory practice is to set a good example.

Chapter 7
Protection from Abuse

Characteristics of abuse and abusers

We have already seen that one of the key duties of a care worker is to protect clients from possible harm. One of the ways to do this is to prevent them from suffering abuse. A distinction is made between the words 'harm' and 'abuse,' because although all abuse is harmful, not all harm springs from abuse.

A carer who loses self control and roughly manhandles a client is both harming the person and subjecting them to physical abuse; a state of affairs that is completely unacceptable. By contrast, clients who are unsteady on their feet and who fall injuring themselves, suffer harm but not necessarily abuse.

From the client's viewpoint, neither situation is satisfactory as both cause injury. The environment they live in should be secure and as free from risk as possible. In addition, the people caring for them should be competent and dedicated to protecting them from harm. Unfortunately, it is impossible to guarantee that accidents will never happen. Abuse is a different matter. Often it is deliberate rather than accidental and, unless it is self-inflicted, it is frequently possible to prevent it.

The media regularly publicises cases of abuse, many of which concern vulnerable people. Children, individuals with learning difficulties and frail elderly people are typical victims. Invariably, the people responsible for abuse are in a close relationship with their victims and sometimes are themselves former casualties of mistreatment.

Abuse comes in many forms. One which causes perhaps the most revulsion is sexual abuse, particularly against children or other susceptible individuals. Physical abuse, where pain or injury is deliberately inflicted upon a victim, also receives wide publicity. Less widely reported are cases of emotional, psychological, verbal or financial abuse in which a victim may be subjected to constant discrimination or humiliation.

In reality, there are no neat divisions between categories of abuse. A physical beating does not simply scar an individual's body, it also injures their mind. The power and control which an abuser wields when physically or sexually assaulting a victim rob that person of their dignity, sense of worth and self-confidence. Similarly, regular attacks of verbal abuse can be just as damaging to an individual as any marks or bruises caused by physical injury. Abusers are not a special class of people. In certain circumstances anyone can be guilty of ill-treating others.

In a famous experiment conducted over 30 years ago, volunteers were duped into believing that by pressing a button they were giving electric shocks to people who had consented to the treatment. The supposed victims were briefed to cry out in agony and beg to have the 'treatment' stopped. Two men dressed as doctors in white coats ordered the volunteers to ignore the protests and increase the strength of the shocks, to make the treatment more effective.

The majority of volunteers taking part in the experiment chose to ignore the victims' screams for mercy. They obeyed the doctors' instructions and many increased the strength of the 'current' to what would have been a lethal level if the electricity supply had been connected.

These experiments set out to discover how far people would go in obedience to authority and group pressure. Their findings appear to indicate that apparently normal individuals can, in certain situations, be guilty of deliberately inflicting pain on vulnerable people.

The discovery in recent years that many elderly people are being abused by members of their own family appears to confirm these findings. The stresses of caring for an elderly parent, without respite, can prove too much for some individuals, especially when the elderly person exhibits difficult or demanding behaviour.

Many carers have gone months without a decent night's sleep. Faced with the almost impossible task of trying to provide twenty-four hour care, some individuals find that they are unable to cope. They reach breaking point and their resulting frustration sometimes spills over into physical abuse.

When this happens, carers who, often unaided, have had to make considerable sacrifices in their own life, can become as much victims as the person they abuse. Many experience tremendous guilt, since most family relationships are based on mutual caring. Individuals are not expected to deliberately inflict pain upon those that they love, even more so if they are frail and elderly.

It can never be justifiable to abuse vulnerable people. Nevertheless, it is wrong to place carers in situations in which they find it impossible to cope. To do so is in itself a form of abuse.

Abuse in residential care

There has been a dramatic increase in the number of recorded instances of abuse in residential care establishments in the public, private and voluntary sectors in recent years. Some doubts exist as to whether this is due to an actual growth in the number of offences, or rather in the amount of cases being reported. Some authorities believe that people are more willing to report abuse, and it is this which accounts for the apparent rise in cases.

A particular cause for concern has been the growth in the number of complaints to the United Kingdom Central Council for Nursing, Midwifery and Health Visiting (UKCC) against qualified nursing staff working in residential nursing homes. The UKCC is the body responsible for maintaining the register for qualified nurses. If complaints about a nurse's conduct are proven, it can lead to the removal of that nurse's name from the register, effectively ending his or her career. According to their own figures, in 1994, cases of complaints involving nursing homes were almost 100% greater than in any other area of practice.

Anxious that residents suffering from debilitating conditions, such as dementia, were unable to complain or represent their own interests, the UKCC issued a report summarising some of the more common complaints of abuse. These ranged from verbal and physical abuse to removing gifts of sweets and food from resident's rooms. Other complaints were:

- administering excessive doses of tranquillisers,
- sleeping on duty,

- leaving residents in soiled beds
- providing inadequate supervision of care assistants.

Social services have also been the subject of a number of complaints and official enquiries, particularly in the area of sex abuse occurring in children's homes. This is why it is necessary for care staff, preferably early on in their training, to have some understanding about the possible causes of ill treatment and how to protect clients from its occurrence.

 Action exercise 7.1 _____

Group discussion:

Is 'verbal abuse' the same as rudeness or 'telling someone off' – if not how does it differ? What effects might regular occurrences of verbal abuse have on the abuser and the person who is subjected to it?

Self-abuse

One of the most distressing forms of abuse is when clients direct it against themselves. Those with severe learning disabilities, or a psychotic illness, are usually the most likely to practise self-abuse, although this is not always so.

Severe forms of self-abuse are comparatively rare. Those afflicted exhibit a range of behaviours almost all of which risk causing some physical injury. Some individuals will scratch themselves until they bleed. Others, left to their own devices, may strike their head against a wall or any nearby sharp object. The resulting injuries rarely have the chance to heal, as the individual often persists in repeating the behaviour. In time, permanent damage becomes apparent as tissue becomes scarred or softened by continual bruising.

Other forms of self-abuse may involve clients in smearing themselves with their own faeces or attempting to eat them. This type of challenging behaviour is even more rare, and individuals seriously affected are likely to be receiving treatment in a specialised unit with appropriately trained staff caring for them.

Nevertheless, there are milder forms of self-abuse which a few clients in residential homes might exhibit. Some may indulge in occasional bouts of self-injury or self-neglect. Usually clients will have a history of challenging behaviour and care staff will be well briefed when taking up post.

The causes of self-injury are not always known. Very occasionally a rare genetic condition can cause affected individuals to behave in this way. Boredom is another possible factor. An environment devoid of adequate interest can induce individuals to seek the sensation of self-stimulation through pain.

Self-abuse is sometimes seen as a form of attention-seeking behaviour, although care needs to be taken with this particular label. Too often it is used in a derogatory way to imply that a client is 'making a nuisance' of themselves. Nevertheless, for a variety of reasons, there are times when clients engage in self abusive behaviour calculated to attract the attention of others.

It may be necessary to refer clients who engage in self-abuse for a psychological assessment. Psychologists can sometimes devise special programmes to treat attention-seeking behaviour.

The treatment of self-abuse is a complex matter and beyond the scope of this book. In reality, care staff will not be left to deal with this problem alone. The involvement of other professionals or agencies will almost certainly be necessary at some point in time. The role of care staff in these matters is to follow the plan of care, and to monitor and record accurately the progress of the client. There may be times when staff have to restrain an individual to stop them from causing themselves serious injury. Care staff may have to give sedative drugs during outbursts of particularly violent behaviour.

To prevent residents from damaging themselves, the application of protective arm splints may sometimes be required. Except in cases of extreme emergency, the use of physical restraints should only be permitted providing appropriate instructions, signed by a person in authority, are written into a client's care plan.

Witnessing self-abuse can be extremely distressing for the staff who have to deal with it, especially for those who are relatively new to the job. Managers should ensure that staff receive proper training to manage situations of self-abuse when they occur and that ongoing support and advice are available.

Another form of self-abuse that is an increasing problem in society is substance abuse. Illicit drugs and alcohol excess affect people of all ages and social classes. Individuals with known problems are unlikely to gain admission to an ordinary residential facility if their addiction is uncontrolled, or if they are not receiving treatment. However, clients may come directly from their home without their problems of addiction being discovered. New clients always require close observation and monitoring to see that they are settling in comfortably, therefore suspicions of substance abuse should quickly become apparent.

The discovery of alcohol or drugs in the client's possession, although not positive proof of addiction, indicates a need for staff to be more vigilant. Other signs that staff should look out for are rapid mood swings, aggressive outbursts and erratic behaviour, all of which can be indications of substance abuse. Carers should immediately report any suspicions that they have to senior staff. The establishment will probably have a system of referral for such clients, which means that, if necessary, they can be given treatment in an appropriate facility.

Injuries and accidents

The best way to protect clients from possible abuse is to prevent it happening in the first place. However, this is not always possible. Consequently, staff have to be alert for any signs of abuse that clients might display, so that it can be dealt with quickly.

Even when care is of the highest standard it is possible for some clients to sustain injuries. Many frail elderly people are unsteady on their feet and can stumble against objects causing bruising or swelling to appear. Accidents of this and a similar nature have to be properly recorded in an appropriate book.

Although it is common policy to record details of accidents, once entered, the information contained within them is often ignored – despite the fact that there can be much to learn from the data. For example, accident reports provide evidence of when and where mishaps occur.

A high level of accidents happening at certain periods throughout the day might indicate that more staff are needed on duty at those times. Alternatively, managers might have to consider the possibility of altering shift patterns to increase staffing during at-risk periods.

Similarly, if a high number of injuries are sustained in a particular area of the home, this might indicate a need for increased observation by staff, or for special adaptations to be installed. Unless staff periodically review the information held in accident reports, they are failing in their duty to provide clients with a secure environment and also flouting the regulations of the Health and Safety at Work Act 1974 which requires such records to be kept.

A significant number of accidents happen in the absence of any reliable witnesses. If a client is confused and unable to explain how they sustained injuries, a report of the accident is still made out, even if its cause is unknown. A large number of accidents occurring apparently unwitnessed should be a cause for concern, particularly if the same staff are on duty at the time. It could indicate that a member of staff was assaulting vulnerable residents. An alternative explanation could be that staff were lax in their observation of clients and should be more vigilant in the future.

Some clients are more accident prone than others, particularly those who have a severe form of epilepsy. Accident records can indicate those who suffer recurring injuries and who may require a change in their medication or need to wear a protective helmet. They may also show that some residents who are unsteady on their feet may benefit by using a walking frame.

The importance of correctly recording details when making out accident reports cannot be overestimated. There is also a need to carry out a regular review of the recorded information. Accident reports, like other forms of documentation, can be required for legal purposes in claims of negligence, or as a statutory requirement under the Health and Safety at Work Act 1974.

Occasionally, staff find themselves involved in court proceedings and any comments they have written in official records are likely to come under close scrutiny. It is therefore essential that details are recorded in a manner that is unambiguous, unbiased and accurate.

 Action exercise 7.2 _____

Discuss potential causes of accidents or health risks which are present in almost everybody's home. What can be done to reduce the chances of accidents happening? What risks (if any) are acceptable to take with vulnerable people living in an ordinary house? For example, should an elderly person of limited mobility and of an independent disposition cook meals for themselves?

Non-accidental injury by clients

Clients, like anyone else, can be guilty of abuse. Unexplained injuries are sometimes discovered on someone sharing a bedroom with another resident. The victim, perhaps through confusion, may have been responsible for night-time disturbances causing their room-mate to lose sleep. Irritability resulting from sleep deprivation can build up to a pitch where an individual loses control and suspicion thus falls upon the room-mate.

If an individual experiences nightly episodes of sleeplessness, there is a real risk that the resulting stress can trigger violence. If staff are suspicious in cases like these, they may have to separate clients or make alternative sleeping arrangements. If the victim sustains no further injuries it is likely that the staff suspicions are justified.

Clients have also been known to exploit other more vulnerable residents. Relationships can spring up in residential homes, particularly between younger members of the client group. Individuals will sometimes want to show their affection by buying a gift for a friend or partner. In most cases this merely mirrors the norms of society. However, there have been instances when a client regularly spends all their spare cash on a 'friend' leaving themselves with virtually nothing.

Staff have a difficult task in circumstances like these. They must satisfy themselves that clients are not coerced into doing something against their wishes. However, they also want to promote the autonomy of clients. It is not an automatic justification for staff to intervene just because someone behaves foolishly. Nevertheless, it is important to establish whether undue pressure is being brought to bear upon an individual. Instances have occurred where clients, particularly those with learning disabilities, have been exploited sexually by their peers, as well as by others. If clients do not give consent for friends or peers to relate to them intimately, then they require the staff to protect them from exploitation. Intimate contact without consent is an assault, and sometimes this point has to be explained to offending clients.

It should be possible, by close observation, to either confirm or rule out regular patterns of abuse by clients. If carers do discover unexplained injuries on an individual, they should carry out regular physical checks. This is to make certain that the resident sustains no further harm. Any examinations should be carried out as discreetly as possible, such as when dressing or bathing a client. Inevitably, observations like these intrude on the privacy of a client, but the greatest priority is to protect them from possible further injury.

On rare occasions visitors and relatives too have been found guilty of abusing clients. When this does occur, it is more likely to happen outside the residential home, either during breaks when a client has gone to stay with relatives, or when taken on a day's outing. All it takes to spark off an aggressive act is a flash of anger, and staff should be aware that visitors are as capable of losing their temper as anyone else.

Signs of abuse

Clients who have difficulty in communicating, such as those suffering from dementia, profound learning disability or psychotic illness, are particularly vulnerable to abuse. They may not be in a position to make their complaints known. Marks or bruising to their bodies may be the first indicators that something is wrong, although abuse can occur even though no injuries are evident. Physical harm does not always leave marks or bruises.

Individuals can be abused emotionally as well as physically. Sometimes staff, for their own perverted amusement, have engaged in constant teasing of a particular individual. Making a client the butt of cruel jokes, or the object of sarcastic remarks, humiliates and belittles them, so too does embarrassing them in front of other people. Comments regarding an individual's shortcomings can lead to an erosion of their self-esteem.

People who indulge in 'winding up' clients in order to deliberately provoke them may have serious problems of their own. The urge to dominate or humiliate others often indicates gross emotional insecurity in an individual's own personality. Fortunately, it is only a very small minority of care staff who set out deliberately to antag-onise clients. However, staff can unintentionally upset the people in their care. Some individuals are more sensitive than others, and an unthinking remark by a carer can sometimes cause them a great deal of distress.

 Action exercise 7.3 _____

One of the characteristics that people often value in others is the ability to laugh at themselves or to 'take a joke'. Discuss the possible reasons for this, and consider how different circumstances may affect people and their ability for self disparagement.

The body language of residents can provide clues to alert staff to possible incidents of abuse. Clients who cower, or show a defensive attitude, may be demonstrating behaviour they have learned in response to acts of aggression. Depression or apathy can be symp-tomatic of learned helplessness where victims submit themselves to situations beyond their control. Fear can sometimes be recognised on the faces of victims and, while not evidence of abuse, it should alert care staff to its possibility.

Other signs that something might be wrong are sudden and drastic changes of behaviour. A normally extrovert client who lapses into quiet apathy might be a victim of ill treatment. Someone who starts indulging in erratic or bizarre conduct may also be a victim of abuse. Although clients with a limited ability to commu-nicate are often at most risk of abuse, articulate clients can also suffer and remain silent. The fear that an abuser is able to generate in a victim can prevent even vocal individuals from making com-plaints. This reinforces the importance of being alert to non-verbal messages given out by clients.

Signs of negligence

A major cause of abuse is negligence and usually there will be physical and psychological signs which accompany this. Under certain circumstances poor health can indicate neglect. Incontinent residents left unattended for hours, for instance, are at risk of developing pressure sores. Lack of mobility, coupled with the effects of incontinence upon the skin, can be particularly damaging to an individual's health; so too can poor nutrition. Clients can become thin and emaciated through negligence. Staff, impatient to press on with their duties, may not allow sufficient time for residents to finish their meals. Half empty plates may be cleared away from clients who are slow to eat their food. Carers can be too preoccupied to notice when a client is not eating normally.

The appetite of residents may be poor because they are depressed or feeling unwell. Sometimes they are simply not receiving sufficient food. Occasionally, some clients will steal food off the plates of their neighbours. If this goes unnoticed, over a period of time, an individual can become seriously malnourished. The resulting weight loss and vitamin deficiencies can have a grave effect on the person's health. Carers have a duty to ensure that clients receive adequate nutrition, and are guilty of negligence if they fail to maintain close observation or control at mealtimes.

Negligence adversely affects the mental as well as the physical health of clients. Residents left sitting for hours deprived of any form of stimulation or activity risk becoming bored and listless. The effect of this mistreatment is that some will lapse into total apathy. Others, in an effort to experience some sensation, may start engaging in self-stimulating behaviour. This can take the form of continuous rocking to and fro, or even, as previously mentioned, incidents of self-abuse.

All human beings need some stimulation from their environment. The inhabitants of a residential home are no different in this respect than anyone else. If they are elderly, they will probably not want to engage in a daily round of energetic activities, but there are a number of things that staff can do to provide an atmosphere that is invigorating. Gentle conversation can be a welcome diversion for some. Others may prefer to go for a walk outside for a change of scenery.

Clients should be encouraged to continue to pursue any existing hobbies or even take up new ones. Most of the scandals that have occurred in long stay institutions over the years have been due to unthinking neglect rather than intentional abuse.

Preventing abuse

Ill health, whether mental or physical, can be due to factors which have nothing to do with abuse. Similarly, the signs described above will not always be caused by mistreatment or negligence. Nevertheless, when seeking explanations of a client's unusual behaviour or physical state, staff should always bear in mind the possibility that it might be related to abuse of some kind.

One of the most effective ways to prevent negligence occurring in the first place is to ensure that quality and standards of care are sufficiently high. Senior staff in particular have a duty to monitor the efficiency and effectiveness of the work of carers to ensure that standards do not fall. Care assistants, however, cannot escape all responsibility for their practice. There will be times when staff are working without supervision, and standards should remain constant even though 'nobody is in charge'.

Managers are busy people. Consequently, there can be times when they are unaware of circumstances that can lead to deficiencies in the quality of care. Staff working directly with clients are likely to be the first to notice if problems affecting care arise. Even in a well-run establishment things can go wrong. Usually maintenance staff will attend to the routine tasks involved in the running of a residential facility, but sometimes jobs that should be done get overlooked.

If this happens, care staff have to do more than just 'soldier on'. Blocked drains and toilets have implications for the health of clients. Similarly, broken locks on doors, or the absence of sufficient screens, adversely affects their rights to privacy. Shortages of staff, due to absence or sickness, are likely to reduce both the quality and quantity of care provision. Employees therefore have a duty to inform or remind managers of service deficiencies, and not simply assume that someone is attending to them. If, despite such warnings, managers fail to act to improve matters, then they themselves are guilty of negligent behaviour.

Many of the cases of negligence which have occurred in the past have been due to staff not being properly trained or inducted into the duties of their new job. Those who did receive some initial training often went many years without it being updated. Or there was a failure to make certain that staff training needs were regularly reviewed.

The advent of nationally recognised qualifications is a vast improvement on what has gone before. However, staff in work have little control over the amount of training they receive. It is left to owners and senior staff to decide who, if anyone, requires to attend further courses. Even when a training deficiency is identified it can be difficult for managers, particularly in small establishments, to release staff from normal duties to further their education.

If staff feel that they are not competent to carry out a specific task because of a lack of training, they must inform their supervisor. Clients are people and not guinea pigs. For instance, if carers have any doubts regarding their ability to tend to someone in the throes of an epileptic seizure, or to assist a colleague in manually handling a resident, then they must refrain from these duties, until they have been trained to undertake them proficiently.

Policies and training

In the past, particularly in long-stay institutions, a number of tragedies have occurred often as a result of insufficient staff training. Residents have been placed by unthinking staff in baths of hot water and scalded to death. Others have died by choking on food which carers should have cut into small portions or liquidised. Some severely confused clients have been left unobserved to wander off into the surrounding countryside. Those inappropriately dressed and not found quickly, sometimes die of hypothermia.

Usually a resident's roaming habits are well known. Individuals at risk, therefore, have to be kept under regular observation. It admittedly can be difficult at times to keep track of clients who suffer from dementia; however, staff have a duty of care towards their clients. Consequently, as well as the need for staff training, policies should exist that deal with the security of the home and residents. In addition, care plans should make it clear whether restrictions should be placed on a client's movements at certain times, for their own safety.

Nursing homes should have other policies to protect clients from possible abuse, such as the safekeeping of personal money or valuables. A number of cases of financial abuse have occurred over the years where staff and relatives have been found guilty of stealing from those in their care. Sometimes vulnerable individuals have been tricked into signing papers giving away their assets, or duped into giving valuables to a carer in the pretence that they are going to be placed in a secure place. Proper receipts should be given to clients for all monies or valuables taken in for safekeeping and full descriptions of properties received should be recorded in an appropriate book. Accountants should have access to these records when undertaking a financial audit.

In every establishment there should also be a procedure whereby clients, or their advocates, can register complaints and be assured that a thorough investigation of their grievances will be undertaken. Policies should be reviewed regularly and updated and staff made aware of any changes or amendments.

Adequate staff training and relevant policies are particularly important when dealing with incidents of aggression. If residents are in danger of being attacked, it is vital that staff act speedily and effectively. Aggression by clients can be directed towards other residents, members of staff or even visitors to the establishment. In all cases staff should summon assistance immediately an incident occurs.

To prevent further injury, it is essential to remove a victim of an assault to a safe place as quickly as possible. This will almost certainly require the assistance of other staff, as while this is being done, someone else will have to talk to the aggressor to prevent them from continuing with their assault.

Separating an aggressor from his or her intended victim is vital, although staff should employ only a minimum amount of force to achieve this. For most people aggressive outbursts are a frightening spectacle. Despite this, staff must remain as calm as possible, or at least give an outward appearance of calm throughout an incident.

Demonstrations of fear or excitement by carers are likely to be communicated to an aggressive client, whose own adrenaline levels will already be high. The key objective for staff is to defuse the situation and pacify the client. This is unlikely to happen if they allow themselves to become overexcited.

Some of the strategies that staff might use to manage disruptive behaviour were discussed in Chapter 3. These range from diverting the attention of the aggressor to implementing a time-out policy. Eventually calm is restored and things return to normal. When this happens, an incident report must be made out and, if injuries are sustained, an accident report.

Following this, staff should try to set time aside to reflect upon the incident. Only by critically discussing it among themselves are they likely to learn anything that might help to prevent a similar event occurring in the future. For instance, were there any advance signs that a client was experiencing a build up of stress? Could staff have been more alert and foreseen the possibility of an outburst occurring? Could staff have dealt with it more quickly or more effectively when violence did erupt? Only by reviewing existing practice is it possible to improve standards of care.

When reviewing an incident of aggression, staff should reflect upon their feelings as well as their actions. It is not uncommon for individuals to experience fear when witnessing a violent outburst, and even more so if it is directed against themselves.

 Action exercise 7.4

List the factors which give rise to feelings of hostility and aggression within yourself. How do you express these feelings (by shouting, throwing objects, hitting out, swearing etc.)? Discuss your feelings immediately after your aggression has subsided. Looking back on an occasion when you lost your temper, was there anything that you could have done to prevent it?

Effects on staff and witnesses

Staff can sometimes experience other powerful emotions, such as anger and resentment, towards an aggressive client, particularly when under stress. These feelings are normal, but carers can be left with a sense of guilt. Others can be emotionally affected by heightened feelings of fear and suffer a loss of confidence in their own ability to cope. It is therefore important for carers to confront their anxieties and tensions by reflecting upon them and, if possible, by talking about them.

Few people will want to reveal much about their private thoughts in a public meeting, but it is helpful if a friend or respected colleague can lend a friendly ear. The importance of peer support is increasingly being recognised as well as the need to establish a network of mutual aid. Peer support usually involves identifying a colleague who is sympathetic, and sharing mutual experiences and concerns. It is not meant to replace advice and assistance, which should be available from senior staff, but rather to complement it.

A violent incident affects bystanders as well as those who are directly involved. Witnesses to violence can react in different ways. Younger people can become stirred up and excitable, even to the extent where they join in. This reinforces the importance of staff dealing with incidents as quickly and calmly as possible.

Frail clients may be particularly anxious when violence breaks out. The sound of raised voices is enough to make some people feel apprehensive, especially if by nature they are timid. People with limited mobility are likely to be fearful if objects are being thrown around and they are caught in the cross-fire. Consequently, once an incident has been dealt with, staff should attend to the needs of those who witnessed it. Almost certainly some will require comforting and reassuring that the incident is over. Once witnesses feel confident enough to talk about their recollections of the incident, they should be encouraged to do so. As well as helping to relieve pent-up stress this may yield useful information to add to an incident report.

The effectiveness with which staff handle incidents of violence adds to the resident's sense of security. An outburst that is mis-handled is likely to leave many feeling uneasy and exposed to potential danger. The regular monitoring of incident reports can provide evidence of whether aggressive outbursts are on the increase. They can also highlight whether some clients are becoming more aggressive.

Sometimes physical conditions, such as the onset of epilepsy or a brain tumour, can be responsible for an individual acting aggres-sively. These possible causes must be ruled out by a medical examination. The aim should be to limit the number of aggressive outbursts to an absolute minimum, thus providing a safe environ-ment in which clients feel secure.

Environmental factors

Environmental conditions affect people's behaviour in different ways. Serious overcrowding, for instance, restricts freedom of movement and can provoke quarrels among people who feel that their personal space is being invaded. Although care homes are unlikely to be overcrowded, staff can get into routines of block treatment which cause too many clients to be in a relatively confined area at the same time.

Some of the worst practices prevalent in long-stay institutions in the past were due to block treatment. During bathing sessions clients awaiting their turn for a bath would often be lined up outside bathrooms. Inevitably, as they milled around bumping into each other in the restricted space, tempers would fray and clashes between residents would occur. Practices like these should no longer exist, but an adverse environment can still be the irritant that causes tensions to rise. This illustrates why incidents must be recorded and reviewed on a regular basis. If there are factors within the environment which provoke disruptive behaviour, they need to be discovered and rectified.

Unwanted noise is increasingly being blamed for many disputes between neighbours living in the community. It can be just as disruptive in a residential home. Sometimes unthinking staff can switch on radios, CD players or televisions and leave them on for hours, regardless of whether anyone is listening. Some clients may not mind too much, while others may experience considerable distress. For clients who are unable to communicate their frustrations by speech, they may resort to exhibiting disruptive behaviour.

In residences where music is selected and played by staff from a central speaker, some thought should be given to the requirements of the audience. Although there will be exceptions, usually elderly folk are unlikely to be eager to listen to the very latest pop music. The music being played should be for the benefit of the residents – not the carers.

It is not only staff who can unwittingly trigger aggressive outbursts. Some elderly clients, with hearing impairments, may operate radios at full volume, which can antagonise those with normal hearing. To reduce the chances of this happening, staff can make sure that individuals with auditory impairments have hearing aids, complete with batteries that work!

Irritations due to lack of stimulation, sleep disturbances, or excessive noise are only a few examples of the many possible ways in which the environment can adversely influence human behaviour.

Therefore, staff have the task of trying to identify those factors in the environment which might be responsible for initiating aggressive outbursts. Unless causes are identified, it is not possible to rectify them and similar incidents are likely to recur in the future. Clients experiencing aggression of any type are being subjected to abuse and the best way to protect them is to provide a rich and satisfying environment.

 Case study

Mr Charlesworth is an elderly gentleman who suffers periodic bouts of paranoia. He believes (entirely without foundation) that staff are telling lies about him, saying that he has a criminal record and that he steals from other residents. Another client, Mr Earnest, who enjoys winding people up, feeds these fantasies by repeating to Mr Charlesworth what staff have supposedly said. How might this situation be dealt with?

Summary of key points

- Abusers are not a special class of people. In certain circumstances anyone can be guilty of perpetrating abuse.
- In the case of self-abuse the role of staff is to follow the plan of care and to monitor and record accurately the progress of the client.
- It should be common policy in residential homes for all accidents to be properly recorded in an appropriate book.
- The information in accident reports should be regularly analysed and reviewed.
- Clients can be guilty of abusing each other. Staff should be aware of this and of the need to keep close observation to either confirm or rule out abuse by clients.
- Marks or bruises are not the only indicators of abuse. Abuse affects people psychologically as well as physically.
- The body language of residents can sometimes provide clues to alert staff suspicions of abuse.
- One of the major causes of abuse is negligence and often there will be both physical and psychological signs which accompany this.

- Employees have a duty to inform or remind managers of service deficiencies, and not simply assume that someone is attending to them.
- If staff feel that they are not competent to carry out a specific task, they must not attempt to do so until they have been trained.
- Staff should remain as calm as possible during an aggressive incident. Their main objectives are to speedily summon assistance, defuse the situation and pacify the client.
- The effectiveness with which staff handle incidents of violence adds to the resident's sense of security. An outburst that is mishandled is likely to leave many feeling uneasy and exposed to potential danger.
- Irritations due to lack of stimulation, sleep disturbances, or excessive noise are some of the ways in which the environment can adversely influence human behaviour.
- Unless the causes of aggression are identified it is difficult to anticipate them and future incidents are likely to recur.

Chapter 8
Whistleblowing

A duty to report

If staff witness incidents in which clients are subjected to abuse they have a duty to intervene. Their obligation to protect clients from harm does not allow them the luxury of 'looking the other way'. Normally, they will report their concerns to their immediate manager, unless it is that individual who is responsible for the ill treatment, in which case it will be to a more senior person. Staff failing to report mistreatment of a client are acting as an accomplice to abuse, morally if not legally.

Unless someone voices their concerns regarding malpractice, it is likely to continue. Once an abuser realises that a witness is not going to report them, there is nothing to stop them continuing with the offences. Furthermore, witnesses who are reluctant to report an incident the first time it occurs, will not find it any easier on other occasions.

A member of staff discovered mistreating a client may plead not to be reported, protesting that it was an isolated incident, a momentary loss of control that they bitterly regret. However, there is no way of knowing if this is true, and abuse, witnessed for the first time, may have occurred on many occasions in the past. One of the golden rules of ethics states that we should treat people the same way that we would like to be treated. Consequently, as few of us are likely to want to be victims of abuse, we should protect others from it.

Care staff have to prevent their clients from suffering harm and to act in their best interests, therefore, to ignore abuse on the grounds of not wishing to become personally involved breaches this fundamental duty.

Apart from duties, there are also rights to consider. Clients have a right to a safe and secure environment and their corresponding responsibilities are to refrain from engaging in activities which endanger the environment for themselves or others.

Abuse is an infringement of human rights, which is why carers have to do everything they can to protect the entitlements of their clients. If staff condone the mistreatment of clients, it follows that they cannot credibly claim to respect them, and treating vulnerable people without respect is a form of abuse. Although the ethical case to report abuse is an overwhelming one, unfortunately many times it still goes unreported.

Reluctance to report abuse

There are historical as well as cultural reasons why staff are often reluctant to report the ill treatment of clients. In long-stay mental institutions in the past, many employees, as well as working together, often lived next to each other too. The hospitals, surrounded by blocks of staff houses, were usually sited in isolated rural areas, the only leisure amenity for miles being the staff social club. Consequently staff often made close relationships as they mixed both socially and in the workplace.

The winding-down of the large mental hospitals put an end to this type of close knit village community. However, despite the more casual relationships that currently exist between work colleagues in residential homes, incidents of abuse still go unreported.

Some of the reasons for this are due to misguided cultural influences. As children we are told not to 'tell tales' or 'sneak' on others. Those who break these taboos are unpopular with their peers and often find themselves ostracised. So strongly ingrained is the perception that it is wrong to inform on others, that even criminals hold in contempt those who 'grass' on their fellows.

Other influences are also at work. In some cases, ignorance and group pressure are to blame. Staff, particularly ones new to the job, may not always realise that it is wrong to shout at residents. If experienced carers set poor examples and spend much of their time yelling at clients, new staff are given poor role models.

If new staff do not know what is a reasonable standard of care, they are unlikely to see anything wrong in unacceptable practices, such as clients being left incontinent for long periods. Fortunately, more staff are now receiving training and the chances of them being unwitting accomplices in mistreating clients are considerably less. However, staff might be aware that standards of care are not as good as they could be, but may be uncertain whether they should report poor practice. Even good staff can have off days, and personal problems or sleepless nights can affect an individual's performance at work.

People are human and mistakes do happen. A potential whistle-blower can find themselves in a dilemma. Do they report a colleague for what might be a solitary lapse from normally high standards? Do they point out to the staff concerned their shortcomings, but stop short of making an official report?

Some things can never be overlooked. Physically striking or sexually abusing a client can never be justified. If there is any risk that the same mistakes, or lapses of standards, will recur in the future, then staff should report their anxieties to someone in authority.

Staff may fail to report abuse because they are not assertive enough. It can be especially difficult for new employees to criticise more experienced carers who have been in post for some time. The tendency to conform to authority and to group pressure has been previously discussed and new employees are more likely to be influenced by these factors. This does not justify staying silent. It simply makes it more difficult to speak out.

Another deterrent to speaking out is victimisation. In the past, people who have had the courage to report wrongdoing have occasionally become victims themselves. Some have been subjected to verbal abuse and received hate mail from colleagues and former friends. Even senior managers have not always been enthusiastic about receiving information concerning deficiencies in the work-place.

There have been instances in commercial firms, where conscience-stricken employees have reported tax-dodging activities to the Inland Revenue. Not only has this resulted in them losing their jobs, but prospective employers have been reluctant to engage such 'Honest Johns', probably because they too have things to hide. In the main, staff working in the care sector have not been so badly treated, although occasionally local unpleasantness has caused employees to leave and seek a fresh start elsewhere.

If people have a family to support and a mortgage to pay, it is not surprising that, at times, they are reluctant to report malpractice. Nevertheless as well as being unethical, it is rarely in their own interests to remain silent. For almost always, the implications of not reporting malpractice are potentially far more damaging to an individual, than any whistleblowing activities.

Loyalty

As mentioned earlier, work colleagues sometimes form attachments with each other making allegations of misconduct especially difficult. Trust and loyalty are the hallmarks of a close personal relationship and whereas people may feel little commitment towards acquaintances or strangers, the same is not true of friends.

People are loyal to their friends. Because they like them, they also make more allowances or excuses for them than for strangers. It is comparatively easy to criticise a person we dislike, or to cause them trouble. It is much harder to do so when dealing with close friends or partners. This does not excuse a failure to report abuse, if the person is someone we know and like. However, it emphasises that witnesses to abuse can face conflicts of conscience that reinforce the need for managers to create a supportive environment for their staff to work in. Enough barriers exist already which make it difficult for carers to express their concerns.

Loyalty is not the exclusive preserve of friends. It is possible to feel loyal towards people we do not especially like, but whom we respect. Managers who do their job competently and who treat people fairly can attract respect from their staff. Indeed, good working relationships between staff and managers depend upon establishing bonds of mutual trust and loyalty.

Dilemmas concerning loyalty can sometimes occur when people have divided loyalties. In the workplace they might have an allegiance to a friend, who is guilty of malpractice, and to a manager who should be informed of the situation. It is not possible in these circumstances to sit on the fence and try to be loyal to both persons: a decision has to be made.

Remaining loyal to the manager by reporting the offence may cost them the friendship of their work colleague, but it protects vulnerable clients. It is also the course of action which brings about the greatest good. The alternative solution betrays the trust of their manager, protects an abuser and damages existing clients as well as possible future ones.

At the very least, witnesses to abuse must tell the abuser that the ill treatment must stop immediately, or they will report matters. If, despite this threat, this has no effect and they continue to stay silent, then their loyalty is misguided and mistaken.

 Action exercise 8.1 _____

Think of someone who is particularly close to you i.e. a friend, relative or partner. Discuss what part loyalty plays in your relationship and what in your opinion would be a breach of loyalty. Consider what circumstances (if any) would convince you not to remain loyal to the wishes of the individual and how you might behave and feel if it was necessary to act against them.

A friend who is an abuser could be acting unintentionally. He or she could be suffering from a mental breakdown which causes them to neglect or mistreat others. Without treatment, the person will remain sick and the abuse is likely to continue. Staying silent does nothing to help the victim or the friend responsible for the suffering. Reporting the friend however, not only puts a stop to the abuse, but also gives him or her the opportunity to receive treatment and get better.

Not all individuals who abuse others are sick. An individual who deliberately abuses vulnerable people, and at the same time compromises a close companion, is not acting as a friend. There are limits to loyalty. It does not demand that we have to accept the behaviour of a friend, regardless of how terrible or harmful it might be.

A carer who intentionally abuses clients is unlikely to be someone with whom many people would wish to make friends. It is possible to befriend someone, only to discover later that they are not the sort of person we originally thought they were. If someone, who we thought was a friend, deliberately abuses other people, they have deceived us about their real character. They would not have been given our trust if we had known their true character. Consequently, any loyalty we continue to show towards them is undeserved. If despite this we remain silent, then loyalty is not being practised as a virtue, but as a convenient excuse not to get involved.

Failing to report abuse

Failure to report abuse is a serious matter which can lead to disciplinary action against staff, or even dismissal. In cases of negligence any individuals who are aware of abuse happening, but who choose to do nothing, are equally likely to be held to blame. In recent years, the public have become much more willing to take their complaints to the civil courts and staff who condone abuse or negligence could find themselves the target of legal action.

To prove negligence three conditions have to be fulfilled. The first condition specifies that an accused person has a duty of care towards the victim. Care workers by the very nature of their job easily satisfy this criterion. Next, it is necessary to prove that negligence has actually occurred. If physical evidence of abuse or negligence is apparent, without any satisfactory explanation to account for it, this may not be too difficult. Finally, it is necessary to show that any damage or harm to an individual is a direct result of the negligent or abusive act.

The standard of proof required in a civil court is considerably less demanding than that of a criminal court, where any reasonable doubts will secure the acquittal of an accused person. Even if negligence is not proved, the stresses of testifying in court and awaiting the court's verdict can be traumatic.

In serious cases of abuse staff can face criminal charges. Witnesses who fail to report abuse in these circumstances can find that their silence has cost them dear, if the police take the view that they have acted as an accomplice in the incident.

Although whistleblowing has sometimes had a temporary adverse effect on the employment prospects of a few individuals, these setbacks have been minor compared to those experienced by employees criticised in reports arising from inquiries into abuse. Usually managers in the care sector will want to know of any malpractice occurring, so that they can stop it at an early stage. Damaging headlines in the local press are the last thing that they want to see. If, despite the silence of witnesses, abuse is revealed, employers will probably want to know why staff refrained from reporting it. In the absence of a satisfactory explanation, it is unlikely that they will want to retain the services of staff they cannot trust.

Perhaps the greatest implication of failing to report abuse is that witnesses to it have to live with their consciences. Even if the mistreatment is never discovered, they will know that they stood by and did nothing while vulnerable people were being systematically abused. They also have to live with the knowledge that their silence means that an abuser is free to continue to inflict even more suffering.

Most people are likely to take into account the seriousness of an offence when considering whether or not to report malpractice. Someone stealing paper clips is committing a wrong but clearly a minor one compared to physically striking a vulnerable resident. This is not to excuse theft. Stealing is a crime regardless of how trivial the worth of the object. Offenders still must be reminded that their actions are wrong and that they risk losing their reputation and job by their behaviour. The discovery of the theft may also place their colleagues under suspicion.

Serious offences of the sort outlined earlier must be reported officially to senior staff. In doing so however, it is vital that witnesses are quite certain of what they have seen. There can be no room for mistakes. It is a cruel breach of ethics to ruin, or cast a slur on, an innocent person's reputation. Even when they are unfounded, allegations often leave the impression that 'there is no smoke without fire'. Too often innocent people are the subject of witch-hunts, merely on the basis of rumour and speculation.

Apart from the misery caused by unfounded allegations, witnesses must be sure of their facts to make certain that any resulting inquiry establishes the guilt of an offender. If a guilty person goes free, they pose a risk to other clients in the future, particularly if they move to a post in another area with a new unsuspecting employer.

Action exercise 8.2 _____

Discuss whether *any* drop in the quality of care should be classified as negligence or not. Identify some possible criteria for deciding what counts as negligence.

Supporting staff

Reporting abuse is undoubtedly a stressful situation, although considerably less so than remaining silent. As well as making statements and being interviewed, at some stage witnesses may have to attend a formal enquiry. This can be nerve racking, not only at the time, but during the waiting period leading up to it.

It is in the interests of managers and owners to promote an environment that encourages staff to report ill treatment and support them when they do. Unless they succeed in this, it is probable that many incidents of abuse will go unreported.

The nature of the working environment is determined by the quality of the relationship that exists between managers and their staff. An atmosphere of trust is essential. Without it, employees are unlikely to pass on sensitive information. Managers need to be approachable and to listen sympathetically. The effectiveness in the way they handle an incident will affect the confidence that staff have in them.

Confidentiality has to be guaranteed in those cases where an employee reports a colleague on the understanding that their own identity will not be disclosed. Witnesses should be informed of their rights. For instance, when they do give evidence at an enquiry, they can usually have a friend, trade union representative or even solicitor present with them.

Often, witnesses who report abuse will at some stage be asked to make a written statement outlining their allegations and to sign a declaration of its truth. At the same time, it should be made clear that they have the option of declining to make a written statement. A refusal to put an allegation in writing undoubtedly makes it extremely difficult for managers to proceed with an investigation into suspected abuse. However, staff may decide that they have salved their consciences and fulfilled their duties by bringing the matter to the attention of senior staff. In these circumstances all that a manager may be able to do, is to monitor closely the suspected abuser. It is not unknown for individuals to make slanderous accusations against innocent people whom they dislike. From a manager's viewpoint, a verbal allegation without a written statement could be just another malicious accusation.

Making a written statement is the most effective way to protect clients from abuse. It also has the benefit of making it clear that the person making the accusation has nothing to hide. Consequently, they are unlikely to find themselves being blamed by an official enquiry, if it finds that a number of staff must bear responsibility for any malpractice.

If a witness is reluctant to make a written statement however, then senior staff should not browbeat them into changing their minds. It is acceptable for supervisors to point out the importance of written evidence and to explain the difficulties of proceeding without it. Ultimately, however, managers have to accept with good grace the final decision of the employee.

Witnesses who experience any verbal or physical abuse from work colleagues as a result of reporting mistreatment have a right to expect protection from senior staff. Managers must act speedily to identify those responsible for the harassment and to discipline or dismiss them, not only for the sake of the witness but also for the clients. Once people become too frightened to report wrongdoing because of possible reprisals against themselves, managers lose control and clients are exposed to a possible reign of terror.

Channels of communication

It is important that whistleblowers make their concerns known to the proper authorities. Normally, as pointed out previously, this will be to their immediate manager. It would be wrong for staff to inform outside agencies of their concerns before first using the normal internal channels of communication. Staff have duties of confidentiality, not only to clients, but to their employers too.

In certain situations it can be a dismissable offence for an employee to reveal confidential information concerning their employer to an outside source. This is important if care staff have signed a contract containing a 'gagging' clause when they took up post. Reporting directly to the press or media is not an option to consider, unless every other avenue to prevent continuing mistreatment has been explored. Apart from betraying the trust of an employer, stories in the local press outlining allegations of abuse are likely to be read by relatives of other clients in the home. Although other clients may not have been mistreated, their relatives could experience unnecessary stress. Relatives may then suffer feelings of guilt at being unable to look after their loved one.

Once the abuse has been reported, if staff find that their immediate supervisor does not pursue the complaint, they should inform the person of their intention to take their concerns elsewhere. If allegations of abuse at any level are being ignored, staff are entitled to pass on their complaints to a higher authority. Usually, it is in the interests of everyone for allegations of abuse to be thoroughly investigated. Nevertheless, exceptions do sometimes occur. If a carer suspects that their concerns are not being dealt with properly within the home, they have a duty to take them to an outside agency, after first informing the most senior person of their intention.

Potential whistleblowers should approach external authorities which monitor the quality of the environment in care establishments. In the case of nursing homes this will be the local health authority. It is responsible for carrying out inspections of nursing homes and would certainly want to know if abuse of clients was deliberately being condoned in any of the establishments within its area.

Residential homes are regulated by a different authority. They are monitored by the registration and inspection unit of the social services. The number should be listed under social services in the local telephone book or the Citizen's Advice Bureau will be able to provide the information.

Concerns about abuse to either authority will be listened to sympathetically. Callers can remain anonymous if they wish and individuals not wishing to speak directly can put their anxieties in writing.

In addition to these outside agencies, a charity called Public Concern at Work (PCAW) has been set up to assist whistleblowers. However, they recommend that people should only approach them after they have first raised the matter with their employer or senior manager. As well as providing support to would-be whistleblowers, this organisation also supplies training to staff in preventing abuse and advice on the content of policies and procedures. Another charitable organisation, Counsel and Care, provides help and advice for people reporting cases of abuse, particularly if they involve elderly people.

Blaming the system

Sometimes mistreatment occurs not directly through the fault of staff but because of deficiencies within the system. The report *Harm's Way* commissioned by the charity Counsel and Care provides a typical illustration.

The report recounts how a daughter visiting her father in a home always seemed to find him wet and smelly. On raising the issue with the matron, she was told that managers had ordered that the number of incontinence pads available to each patient per day must be restricted.

The matron went on to explain that the managers were forced to make this decision, as there had been a change in the policy of the local health authority. Previously they had supplied incontinent pads free, or at a discount, to private nursing homes but now this was to end.

Some sympathy has to go to managers and administrators who, when funding or resources are cut, are still expected to maintain the same quality of service. There are times when it becomes impossible to make further savings without adversely affecting care practices. However, it is never acceptable to allow vulnerable clients to sit around in urine or faeces-soaked clothes, regardless of what savings have to be made. In a situation like this, it is still necessary to report poor quality of care. Care staff should report that reducing the number of incontinence pads is having a detrimental effect on client care. The matron has to pass this information on to her managers. In all probability this was what happened.

Owners and senior managers must be involved in the reporting process too. They may have to refer matters to the local MP and even enlist the evidence and support of the daughter who raised the matter in the first place. If other relatives are made aware of the policy regarding incontinence pads, they too may be encouraged to bring their concerns to their local health authority, MP or the press.

Senior managers may not be in a position to prevent cuts to services, but they can make known their concerns to influential people. Due to their relatively powerful influence compared to direct care staff, senior managers are in a far better position to protest at unreasonable budgetary restrictions that cause an unacceptable lowering of care standards. Simply blaming the system without making any attempt to improve matters is a convenient excuse for doing nothing.

Witnessing malpractice and failing to intervene to stop or report it, is as blameworthy as actually abusing someone. No matter what the difficulties may be, it is never justifiable to ignore mistreatment.

 Case study

Your senior manager calls you into the office and says that a member of staff has made a complaint against you. The person alleges that you are verbally abusing some of the more difficult older clients by continually shouting at them and some of them are frightened by this. You agree that you have had to raise your voice to one or two clients, but only because they are hard of hearing. In your own mind you know that you have never deliberately abused any of the clients. Discuss how you feel about this accusation, how you would explain your actions and why you think the accusation was made in the first place. Then consider the situation from the manager's viewpoint and discuss how he or she might deal with the situation.

Summary of key points

- If staff witness incidents in which clients are being abused they have a duty to intervene to protect them.
- The implications of not reporting malpractice are potentially far more damaging to an individual, than any whistleblowing activities.
- Loyalty to a friend is not an acceptable reason for refraining from reporting mistreatment.

- Failing to report abuse is a serious matter which can lead to disciplinary action, dismissal or even legal action being taken against an individual.
- It is vital that witnesses are not mistaken and are quite certain of what they have seen. It is unethical to make unfounded allegations against an innocent person's reputation.
- It is in the interests of managers and owners to promote an environment that encourages staff to speak out against ill treatment and support them when they do.
- When asked to make a written statement, staff have the option of declining to do so.
- Staff should report their concerns to their immediate manager. It is wrong to inform outside agencies before using the normal internal channels of communication.
- Staff have duties of confidentiality to their employers as well as to their clients.
- If staff feel that abuse is not being dealt with properly in an establishment they have a duty to take their concerns to an outside agency, after first informing managers of their intention.

Chapter 9

Ethics in the Workplace

Ethics in the working environment

In the preceding chapters the focus has been on the interests of clients. As vulnerable people they have priority over others, especially as staff have a duty of care towards them. However, ethics concerns itself with how we *ought* to treat all people – including the staff.

The ethical principles involved in keeping promises, telling the truth, treating people fairly and respecting them as individuals apply as much to employees as to clients. Unfortunately, abuse of workers is on the increase. Cases of sexual harassment, racial discrimination and bullying in the workplace have all been widely publicised in recent years.

Managers and staff in senior positions are sometimes responsible for these unacceptable practices, but not always. As previously stated, workers who have been courageous enough to blow the whistle on dubious practices have sometimes been persecuted by their own colleagues.

If care workers are treating each other without respect, there is a danger that they will treat clients in a similar manner. In addition, the quality of care is unlikely to improve if morale is low due to poor treatment of staff by managers or colleagues. Not only is it unethical to mistreat fellow workers, it is also an ineffective way to provide health and social care.

Staff who are unfairly treated by being overworked or by receiving insufficient training face enormous stresses. Sickness rates can increase along with the likelihood of making serious mistakes. The turnover of staff in poor working environments tends to be high, which adds to recruitment and training costs, and in turn leads to less money being spent on client care. A constant influx of new staff makes it difficult to build an effective working team that practises a consistent standard of care. All these factors have a direct implication for the client group, as well as for the staff themselves.

Senior staff have an important part to play in workplace ethics. The examples they set will influence the way that employees under their supervision behave. A senior member of staff is in no credible position to rebuke others about poor timekeeping, if their own punctuality is poor. If a supervisor is constantly late on duty they are giving out a message to other staff that punctuality is unimportant. Similarly, if they are abrupt with clients, appear to be workshy or in the habit of gossiping about other people, then they are not acting as appropriate role models. Employees at all levels, not just managers, set the examples for new staff to follow. If the standards set are poor, they are likely to remain so, as new workers copy them and settle into their posts.

Supervisors are usually responsible for making out shift duties and staff rotas. These need to be made out both fairly and efficiently. If employees feel that some staff receive special treatment when it comes to asking for certain days off, it is likely to lead to resentment among members of the team. Rotas should ensure that enough staff are on duty so that carers have as much support as possible when working. Nobody should be left to work with insufficient back up, except in cases of genuine emergency.

Managers should institute performance review or appraisal systems so that staff receive feedback on their overall progress. Appraisal interviews also give staff an opportunity to discuss their own needs regarding the job and any concerns they may have.

As well as an annual system of review, it is important for managers to create a climate where staff feel free to approach them for advice and support. However, staff themselves also have to take responsibility for establishing an ethical environment in the workplace.

Staff responsibilities

Ethics is not just about theories, rules and principles, neither is it a topic that is just relevant to academics, philosophers and other people. It is the concern of every one. It does not demand that people become paragons of virtue, nor can it solve all the problems and dilemmas which individuals come up against. What it can do in the workplace is to improve relationships and contribute towards creating a positive environment. For that to happen, everybody has to make an effort to consider other viewpoints and reflect on their own practice.

The attitudes people have towards their work is influenced by the quality of the relationships they enjoy with their colleagues. Even if their relationship with their boss is not good, it probably affects them less than a poor relationship with a colleague.

Managers have a range of duties to carry out which differ from those of the people under their control. Most of the time employees are not working as closely with their supervisors as they are with their co-workers. Consequently, there is little chance of them avoiding interaction with each other.

People are unique and have a variety of different characteristics. Usually they will get on better with individuals who share the same values, attitudes or interests as themselves. There will be others they meet whom they neither like nor dislike, and inevitably there will be some with whom they have nothing in common. Ethics is concerned with interacting with all people regardless of whether they are friends or not.

Staff have a responsibility to try to get on in the working environment for the sake of clients, as well as for themselves. An environment which is poisoned by malice is not a happy place either to work or reside in.

The way in which people communicate has much to do with the quality of their relationship. Listening is particularly important. It is the most effective way to find out what another individual thinks and feels; it helps people to understand the behaviour of others. Talking is important too, providing that conversation does not centre exclusively upon the needs of the person speaking. Whether we have a genuine concern in the interests of others or not, it costs nothing to be polite and ask people to talk about things that matter to them.

When people show concern for each other, it usually leads to an increase in mutual liking and respect. Praising one another is also beneficial. Carers have little difficulty in praising the efforts of their clients, but with colleagues it is often different. While staff are quick to point out the mistakes and omissions which fellow workers are guilty of, they seldom reward good work or helpful assistance with praise. This may be due to cultural factors that cause people to feel embarrassed when giving out compliments. Nevertheless, individuals have to overcome this obstacle if they are to successfully achieve better working relationships.

There are times when even the best of friends or partners fall out and exchange angry words. Those who really value their friendship, or the relationship they have with a partner realise that someone must make the first move at reconciliation. Marriages and partnerships have to be worked at, and sometimes having to say sorry is necessary if quarrels are to be resolved.

If individuals only consider events from their own perspective, it prevents them from being able to compromise. It also makes reconciliation difficult. At times, it is predictable that other people will treat us unfairly or without respect; everyone is guilty of this and is prone to making mistakes about the actions of other people.

The tendency is for individuals to interpret the behaviour of others in terms that relate to themselves. The motorists on the road ahead of us who fail to indicate are careless. However, it is unlikely that they are setting out deliberately to antagonise us. Similarly, people we know who ignore a cheery greeting may genuinely not notice us, or be too lost in their own thoughts to respond. It does not necessarily mean that they are snubbing us.

In the workplace much backbiting can occur because employees wrongly interpret the behaviour of colleagues. A carer who fails to do a job properly may not be lazy, but simply unaware of his or her own shortcomings. Moaning and grumbling about an individual leads nowhere except to an unhappy working environment. Staff have a duty in such cases to explain and, if necessary, demonstrate the best way to undertake the particular task.

However situations are different if, despite any help, someone chooses deliberately not to work in the required manner. Action is necessary, and if other employees share the same opinion, they should speak out. Unless there is an immediate improvement in performance, they should inform the person concerned that they will report their grievances to a senior member of staff.

Action exercise 9.1 _____

Discuss the factors that make up a satisfactory relationship with work colleagues and identify circumstances that can adversely affect it.

Complaints

One of the most difficult things is to see an issue from another person's point of view. Nevertheless, we have to make an effort to try and understand the ideas and beliefs of others. Empathy, or the practice of putting oneself into another person's position, is a valuable asset for anyone to cultivate. In some situations it can help to reduce the effects of both prejudice and anger.

Sometimes, clients or visiting relatives may complain at what they perceive to be poor standards of care. Regardless of whether or not a complaint is justified it must be attended to promptly. If it is ignored, or dismissed as being trivial, the likelihood is that the person making the complaint will become angry. Trying to see things from the other person's perspective can help prevent losing one's own temper.

It never pays to start arguing with someone who is already angry. They are not going to listen to what is being said, and instead it is better to try calming them down. This may entail offering an apology, even though the incident which has upset them is not the fault of the staff. Naturally if the complaint is justified and you are the person responsible, an apology is required anyway. An assurance that the offence will not be repeated in the future will also be needed.

When it is someone else's fault, or the complaint is unjustified, apologising to someone because they are upset is not necessarily an acceptance of blame. However, by extending sympathy it avoids needless confrontation. Any apology has to be speedily followed with the promise to immediately bring the matter to the attention of a senior member of staff to ensure that appropriate action is undertaken. Unless it is a very minor matter, the person making the complaint will demand to see someone in authority anyway, but as it is the care staff who are usually the first people to receive a complaint, it is essential that they demonstrate a receptive attitude. This means listening carefully to what is being said, clarifying any uncertainties and reporting the incident promptly, while at the same time remaining courteous! Not all complaints will be justified and sometimes this will have to be pointed out diplomatically. However, this task is better left to the supervisor or senior manager, as it is unlikely that a client or visitor will want to be told that they are mistaken, or in the wrong, by a comparatively junior member of staff.

Bullying and harassment

Some managers have come under increasing criticism for the persistent bullying of employees in the workplace, although bullying and harassment are by no means confined to managers and supervisors. Workmates have also been guilty of intimidating colleagues. Some employees, not wanting to be labelled as 'blacklegs' by their fellow workers, have been coerced into joining in industrial action against their wishes. Others have been intimidated into keeping silent about illegal activities such as pilfering by fellow employees, or compelled to participate in dubious practices such as 'clocking on' absent colleagues.

Victims of bullying have increasingly been prepared to give testimony against their tormentors in the form of racial or sexual harassment. In some cases, employers have had to pay substantial damages resulting from awards made by industrial tribunals or civil courts.

Bullying comes in many forms. Besides intimidation, it includes verbal abuse or making offensive remarks. A fine line exists between playful teasing and comments calculated to hurt or humiliate. What one individual may see as a joke another might regard as an insult.

Some people may be appear to be unduly sensitive to what others consider to be harmless remarks. However an individual's early experiences affects them significantly. If in the past they have been the butt of racial, ageist or religious insults it is hardly surprising if they are suspicious of certain nicknames or jokes.

The same may be true of other characteristics. Not every tall person enjoys being addressed as 'lofty', anymore than someone with red hair wants to be known as 'ginger' or 'carrots'. Addressing fellow employees in the manner they prefer is just as important as it is for clients. To knowingly call someone by a name they find offensive is a form of bullying.

Action exercise 9.2 _____

Identify different types of bullying and discuss possible reasons to account for them. Discuss also what methods might be effective in dealing with people who bully.

If doubts exist as to whether someone is likely to be upset by an intended humorous remark, it is best to refrain from making it. This does not mean that joking is wrong. Nobody wants to work in an atmosphere of gloom, fearful of saying anything that might upset another individual. It is not unethical to have fun and enjoy oneself, providing that we are sensitive to the feelings of others.

Without humour, work can be a very dull place. A little light-hearted chat, both with clients and colleagues, improves morale and makes for a happier environment. So too does building relationships and getting to know our workmates. If we succeed in this, we will quickly find out their likes and dislikes – what offends and pleases them. After all if someone tells a risqué joke, it is hardly likely that they will find offence if one is told back to them.

Competence

Carers have to be competent in what they do and this places a number of duties both upon themselves and their supervisors. Staff new in post must not be left alone or 'thrown in at the deep end'. Supervisors should make sure that either they, or an experienced colleague, work closely with inexperienced employees. From a legal viewpoint, a supervisor who leaves an inexperienced member of staff to work unsupported could face serious charges if an accident resulting in injuries occurred.

Apart from initial training, employers should try to ensure that staff also receive ongoing education. Policies and procedures change and staff have to be up to date, particularly if knowledge concerning new treatments or care practices becomes available.

Employees also have ethical responsibilities regarding training. If an employer is paying for a carer to attend a course or study day, then there is a corresponding duty for an employee to improve their performance as a result of their increased knowledge. Ongoing training is ultimately meant to benefit the client. Attending a study day may be a pleasant break from one's usual job, but employees have duties to do much more than merely attend.

Concentration has to be given to what is being taught. This includes asking questions if some things are unclear and not sitting in silent ignorance, above all trying to put into practice what has been learned in theory. There may be an opportunity for the care worker to prove their competence and thus obtain a vocational qualification at some time in the future.

In order to be competent, carers have to take some responsibility for their own learning. Employers cannot always afford to release staff for further training. Sometimes, one member of staff will be released and it will be their responsibility to pass on their new-found knowledge to other team members. This they should do, to the best of their ability. In the absence of formal study periods staff should try to update their knowledge by their own efforts. This may entail reading specialist magazines or articles in newspapers concerning items related to their work, or reading policy documents relevant to the place where they work. It may mean asking more experienced workers for advice, support or even their opinions. There is a duty, regardless of whether an employer supplies training or not, for a care worker to become as competent as they can.

Apart from any ethical considerations, employees have legal duties under the Health and Safety at Work Act 1974 to work in a safe manner and not endanger themselves or anyone else. Ignorance of a procedure is not a defence that will allow them to escape all responsibility, if their actions cause injuries to others.

The requirement not to treat clients as guinea pigs by carrying out procedures which staff have not been trained to do, has already been discussed. Equally important is not to deliberately conceal one's ignorance from colleagues. If asked for advice, it is essential to admit to a lack of knowledge. If ignorant of the correct response, making a wild guess on what to do is not an acceptable option.

Reducing stress at work

A number of times throughout this book the importance of asking senior staff for support has been mentioned. Unfortunately, some people are still reluctant to ask for help, because they mistakenly believe it to be a sign of weakness. Instead they soldier on, in the deluded belief that by not troubling their manager they are some-how proving their competence.

Managers are busy people and sometimes may appear to be too preoccupied to offer help when it is needed. Despite this, staff should not proceed with any care or treatment if they do not feel competent to do so.

If a supervisor is too busy to help, or not immediately available, it may be necessary to alter priorities. Most routine tasks can be put on hold until someone with experience is available to help. In the event of genuine emergencies arising, there should be appropriate policies outlining what actions to take.

Carers have a duty to inform their supervisor if they are working in conditions of undue stress. Temporary staff shortages in the workplace are almost unavoidable, but nobody should have to work in impossible conditions. Usually, employers will be aware of any difficulties that staff face in carrying out their duties. Never-theless, it will do no harm to bring unsatisfactory conditions to their attention.

Employees have a right to protection from assault by clients. At job interviews it should be explained if any duties include looking after clients who can be aggressive. While any potential risks should be put into perspective and not overexaggerated, they should nevertheless be discussed, as well as the support mechanisms that are available to staff who have to deal with violence.

It is of little help to managers if staff become ill as a result of work-related stress. Their absence from duty will only make matters worse for the remaining staff, and for clients too. Employers can be held legally accountable for failing to alleviate unreasonable levels of stress in the workplace. In addition, staff are also more likely to make mistakes when working under stressful conditions.

If employees do make mistakes, they have a duty to report them to their supervisors. There is no point in attempting to conceal errors in the hope that they will never be discovered. Lying or deliberately concealing matters is unethical for a number of reasons. In the first place, it betrays a trust between an employee and an employer: neither expects the other to lie to them. Secondly, a mistake which is discovered, but not admitted to, places unfair suspicion upon colleagues. Even more seriously, it can endanger the welfare of clients. Mistakes are both predictable and stressful, consequently managers should try to create a climate where staff feel they will be treated reasonably if they admit to errors.

The UKCC were concerned that managers were unjustly disciplining nurses who made mistakes in drug administration and circulated a memorandum offering advice. It pointed out that nurses who commit errors should not automatically be disciplined but cautioned instead, and if necessary given additional training. The UKCC were worried that nurses would fail to report their mistakes if it automatically put their careers in jeopardy. The UKCC were careful to point out that disciplinary action should be taken against nurses who made repeated mistakes, or ones that gravely affected the well-being of patients.

This does not mean that managers must overlook carelessness, or not caution care workers about their future conduct. It does mean however, that they should make sure that staff receive a fair and sympathetic hearing and also take measures to ensure that mistakes are avoided in the future.

Morale and recruitment

The principle of respect applies as much to staff as it does to clients. Poor timekeeping, even if it goes unnoticed by a supervisor, will be resented by colleagues. While anyone can be late occasionally, someone who makes a habit of it is showing a disregard for the feelings and needs of colleagues. In addition, they are treating them unfairly. If someone is late, staff are left to carry on working short-handed while clients have to wait longer to be attended to. Similarly, there should be fairness in sharing out tasks. Nobody wants to carry someone on their team who is not prepared to do a fair day's work.

For standards of care to remain high it is important that staff work well together. Good teamwork is essential. Unfair practices by individual workers erode team spirit in the same way that petty squabbles do. Supervisors as team leaders must ensure that differences between personnel are quickly resolved. If personality clashes are too pronounced, employees may have to be separated to work on opposing shifts.

To a large extent, senior staff will determine the morale and motivation of team members. If they take a genuine interest in the things that concern their staff, and treat them fairly, this will go a long way in creating an enjoyable working environment. Favouritism of any kind is likely to cause resentment and lower morale. Poor communication between managers and staff hinders the establishment of good teamwork and so too does constant criticism in the absence of any praise.

Clients, particularly vulnerable ones, have a right to be cared for by staff who are both competent and well-motivated. Until recently there was no national register for care staff, but in 1991 Susan Brooks founded the National Register for Carers (NRC) based in Liverpool. The register records previous employment details and any professional qualifications such as National and Scottish Vocational Qualifications. The decision for carers to register is a voluntary one at present, but as employers increasingly realise the benefits of employing staff who have been thoroughly vetted, applications for registration are likely to expand in the future. The NRC also offers advice and training at various levels to members and will act on complaints made concerning allegations of abuse.

As yet there is no universally agreed Code of Conduct for care workers and this may be the next step in the search for improving care practices in residential homes.

It is vital that managers recruit the right calibre of staff to work with vulnerable people. References should be scrupulously checked and any missing gaps in the employment history of an applicant satisfactorily accounted for.

When giving references to employees who are leaving, it is essential that they represent a true reflection of the person's character. If someone is clearly unsuitable to work as a care assistant, it is morally wrong to provide them with a reference recommending them for another post. If an undesirable employee is taken on by an unsuspecting manager in another area, it shows a scant disregard for the needs of clients. A manager does not have to provide a reference to a departing employee. If an ex-employee is unsuitable to work as a care assistant, sometimes the best policy is to decline to provide a reference for such a post.

Once recruited, staff have a duty to care for the clients to the best of their ability. If they do find that after an initial settling in period they do not like the job, or are unsuited to it, then they should leave. It is better both for them and for their clients to do so. There are times when the most ethical thing that an individual can do, is to simply make sure that they are working in the right job.

 Case study

Mrs Day is a very experienced care assistant who works on the same shift as yourself. You and your colleagues resent the fact that she appears to do far less work than the rest of you. She often spends a long time talking to clients at busy times of the day instead of getting on with the work. She often slips out to have a quick smoke in the staff room even when it is not an official break time. She appears to be on good terms with the supervisor who has worked with her for many years. How might you (or your colleagues) deal with this situation?

Summary of key points

- The ethical principles involved in keeping promises, telling the truth, treating people fairly and respecting them as individuals apply as much to staff as they do to clients.
- If care workers are treating each other inappropriately, there is a danger that they will treat clients in a similar manner.
- Employees set examples for new staff to follow. If the standards set are poor, they are likely to remain so in the future, as the new workers settle into their posts.
- Ethics can improve relationships and contribute towards creating a positive environment in the workplace.
- Listening to people improves the quality of the relationship between them.
- Staff are often quick to point out the mistakes and omissions which fellow workers make and seldom reward good work with praise.
- One of the most difficult things is to see something from another person's point of view.

- Direct care staff are usually the first people to receive a complaint. It is essential that they demonstrate a receptive attitude by listening carefully, clarifying any uncertainties and reporting the incident promptly.
- If there are any doubts as to whether someone is likely to be upset by a humorous remark, it is best to refrain from making it.
- Supervisors, or an experienced colleague, should work closely with inexperienced staff.
- When attending training sessions, staff should concentrate on what is being taught, ask questions if they do not understand and try to put into practice some of the things that they have learned.
- Staff have a duty to inform their supervisor if they are working in conditions of undue stress.
- Managers need to create a climate where staff feel they will be treated reasonably if they admit to making mistakes.
- Good teamwork is essential if standards of care are to remain high.
- If staff find that they are not suited to a post as a care assistant then they should leave.

Further Reading

British Medical Association (1995) *The Older Person: Consent and Care*, London: BMA.

Counsel and Care (1995) *Care Betrayed*, London: Counsel and Care.

Counsel and Care (1997) *Harm's Way*, London: Counsel and Care.

Department of Health (1993) *Guidance for Staff on Relations with the Public and Media*, London: HMSO.

McMahon, C. & Harding, J. (eds) (1994) *Knowledge to Care: a handbook for care assistants*, Oxford: Blackwell Science.

McMahon, C. & Isaacs, R. (1997) *Care of the Older Person: a handbook for care assistants*, Oxford: Blackwell Science.

Nazarko, L. (1996) *NVQs in Nursing and Residential Homes*, Oxford: Blackwell Science.

Nazarko, L. (1995) *Nursing in Nursing Homes*, Oxford: Blackwell Science.

Royal College of Nursing (1992) *Focus on Restraint* (second edition), London: RCN.

Rowson, R.H. (1990) *An Introduction to Ethics for Nurses*, London: Scutari Press.

Stockwell, F. (1972) *The Unpopular Patient*, London: RCN.

Tschudin, V. (1992) *Values Workbook A Primer for Nurses*, London: Baillière Tindall.

United Kingdom Central Council For Nursing, Midwifery and Health Visiting (1994) *Professional Conduct – Occasional Report on Standards of Nursing in Nursing Homes*, London: UKCC.

Useful Addresses

Action on Elder Abuse
1268 London Road
London SW16 4ER
Tel: 0181 679 2648

Age Concern England
Astral House
1268 London Road
London SW16 4ER
Tel: 0181 679 8000

Carers National Association
22–25 Glasshouse Yard
London EC1A 4JS
Tel: 0171 490 8818

CARE
13 Harwood Road
London SW6 4QP
Tel: 0171 371 0118

Counsel And Care
Twyman House
16 Bonny Street
London NW1 9PG
Tel: 0171 485 1550

Help the Aged
16–18 St James Walk
London EC1R 0BE
Tel: 0171 253 0253

Mencap
123 Golden Lane
London EC1Y 0RT
Tel: 0171 454 0454

MIND
15–19 Broadway
London E15 4BQ
Tel: 0181 522 1728

National Register for Carers
PO Box 335
Liverpool
L69 7PA
Tel: 0151 707 9996

Patients Association
18 Victoria Park Square
London E2 9PF

Public Concern at Work
Lincoln's Inn House
42 Kingsway
London WC2B 6EN
Tel: 0171 404 6609

Registered Nursing Home
  Association
Calthorpe House
Hagley Road
Edgbaston
Birmingham B16 8QY
Tel: 0121 454 2511

Relatives Association
5 Tavistock Place
London WC1H 9SS
Tel: 0171 916 6055

SANE (Mental Health Charity)
199–205 Marylebone Road
London NW1 5QP
Tel: 0171 724 8000

The Commission for Racial
  Equality
Elliot House
10/12 Allington Street
London SW1E 5EH
Tel: 0171 828 7022

Glossary

Advocacy Speaking out to secure rights and safeguard interests either for oneself or for another person or group.

Anti-convulsant A drug used in the treatment of epilepsy.

Autonomy The freedom to make one's own decisions and determine one's own course of action.

Block treatment The practice of treating clients in groups regardless of their individual needs.

Care plan An agreed plan of action to meet the needs of an individual client produced after consultation and discussion with clients, relatives, professional staff and colleagues.

Challenging behaviour Behaviour displayed by clients which is detrimental to their best interests and challenges staff to teach alternative positive behaviour.

Code of conduct A document outlining some key principles of how a member of a profession ought to act towards the clients he or she serves.

Distributive justice Seeking, when resources are scarce, the fairest way to allocate goods and services.

Ethical dilemma Uncertainty regarding which is the best moral decision to take, because of conflicting reasons.

Ethical principles A number of ethical rules which can be used as a justification for taking certain moral decisions or actions.

Ethics A branch of philosophy concerned with right and wrong. It focuses upon how people ought to behave towards each other.

Gagging clause A stipulation inserted into an employment contract which prohibits employees from discussing or writing about events related to their work outside their place of employment.

Hallucination A mistaken idea due to the apparent perception of an external object when no such object is present.

Harm principle A justification for overriding an individual's choice of action in order to prevent it from harming others.

Impairments of autonomy Barriers which inhibit the ability to make decisions for oneself.

Informed consent The giving of voluntary consent without any form of coercion and having enough knowledge and comprehension of the subject to make an enlightened decision.

Institutionalisation The routine and uniform treatment of people as a group which causes them to lose their individuality.

Learned helplessness A passive acceptance of one's fate due to being in the control of others and powerless to change things.

Moral rights A justified entitlement to have or do something such as the right to a freedom of speech.

Paranoia A mental disturbance which causes an individual to experience feelings of persecution.

Paternalism Overriding an individual's autonomy by making decisions on their behalf in the interests of their own welfare.

Placebo A harmless substance given to someone who believes they are receiving an authentic medicine.

Positive discrimination Favouring disadvantaged people over the rest of society by an uneven distribution of goods or provision of increased opportunities.

Principles of normalisation A philosophy which focuses on supporting vulnerable people to live culturally valued lives.

Psychotic Disturbed mental behaviour in which the individual has no insight into their condition.

Respect for persons A principle emphasising the unique properties and values placed on human life compared to those placed on non-human organisms.

Stereotype Generalisations which categorise people into groups according to assumed common characteristics.

Stigma A label attached to an individual branding them as unworthy or inadequate.

UKCC The United Kingdom Central Council for Nurses, Midwives and Health Visitors, the statutory body responsible for holding the register for these professional staff.

Utilitarianism An ethical theory based on the belief that one should always act to secure the greatest happiness for the greatest number.

Veracity   Truthfulness – absence of deceit.

Victimisation   The process of unfairly discriminating against someone by making them a scapegoat.

Index

abuse
  by clients, 100–101
  characteristics of, 93
  preventing, 98, 104–5
  self abuse, 96–8
  signs of, 101–3
Access to Health Records Act, 68
accidents, 73, 93, 98–9
advocacy, 52–4
aggression
  and staff training, 106
  as challenging behaviour, 25
  reporting, 14
  responses to, 102
attention seeking, 29, 97
authority
  and complaints, 121
  as power, 1
  conforming to, 114
  obeying, 94
  parental, 10
  signed, 97
autonomy
  as freedom, 12–13
  over-ruling, 24
  promoting, 21, 24, 53, 100
  stifling, 27, 53

behaviour
  challenging, 25, 39–42, 97
  changes, 102
  effects of environment, 108–10,
  erratic, 98
  influence of beliefs, 9–10, 27
  labelling, 29
  negligent, 104
  of clients, 86, 91

  of staff, 81–2, 86
  patterns, 15, 63, 88
  prohibiting, 24
  sexual, 66
beliefs
  and behaviour, 6–7
  and discrimination, 83
  and identity, 4
  harmful, 22
  of conscience, 11
body language, 49, 81, 102

care plan, 91, 97, 105
codes of conduct, 11, 22
communication
  and institutionalisation, 45, 53
  and normalisation, 51–2
  and trust, 53
  barriers to, 48–9
  by touch, 50–51
  channels of, 120–22
  effective listening, 54–5
  skills, 13
  systems, 52–3
community
  and values, 8
  care in the, 77
  close knit, 113
  conflicts within, 21, 86
  disputes, 109
  moving into, 29, 37
competence, 131–2
complaints
  dealing with, 83, 87, 129–30
  legal action, 117
  procedures, 106
  to UKCC, 95–6